Oxford Specialist Handbooks in Cardiology
Adult Congenital Heart Disease

Second Edition

Edited by

Sara Thorne
Queen Elizabeth Hospital
Edgbaston
Birmingham, UK

and

Sarah Bowater
Queen Elizabeth Hospital
Edgbaston
Birmingh;

T0177541

OXFORD
UNIVERSITY PRESS

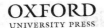

OXFORD
UNIVERSITY PRESS

Great Clarendon Street, Oxford, OX2 6DP,
United Kingdom

Oxford University Press is a department of the University of Oxford.
It furthers the University's objective of excellence in research, scholarship,
and education by publishing worldwide. Oxford is a registered trade mark of
Oxford University Press in the UK and in certain other countries

Published in the United States of America by Oxford University Press
198 Madison Avenue, New York, NY 10016, United States of America

British Library Cataloguing in Publication Data

Data available

Library of Congress Control Number: 2017935050

ISBN 978–0–19–875995–9

Printed and bound in Great Britain by
Ashford Colour Press Ltd.

Oxford University Press makes no representation, express or implied, that the
drug dosages in this book are correct. Readers must therefore always check
the product information and clinical procedures with the most up-to-date
published product information and data sheets provided by the manufacturers
and the most recent codes of conduct and safety regulations. The authors and
the publishers do not accept responsibility or legal liability for any errors in the
text or for the misuse or misapplication of material in this work. Except where
otherwise stated, drug dosages and recommendations are for the non-pregnant
adult who is not breast-feeding

Links to third party websites are provided by Oxford in good faith and
for information only. Oxford disclaims any responsibility for the materials
contained in any third party website referenced in this work.

Contents

Part 1 Introduction to adult congenital heart disease

Part 2 Specific lesions

Part 3   General management issues of adult congenital heart disease

Detailed contents

Symbols and abbreviations

➔	cross reference
↑	increased
↓	decreased
→	leading to
♂	male
♀	female
+ve	positive
−ve	negative
±	with or without
2D	2-dimensional
3D	3-dimensional
6MWT	6-minute walk test
AA	ascending aorta
ACEI	angiotensin converting enzyme inhibitor
ACHD	adult congenital heart disease
AD	autosomal dominant
AF	atrial fibrillation
ALS	advanced life support
Ao	aorta
A-P	antero-posterior
AP	aortopulmonary
AR	aortic regurgitation or autosomal recessive
ARB	angiotensin receptor blocker
AS	aortic stenosis
ASD	atrial septal defect
AT	anaerobic threshold
ATP	anti-tachycardia pacing
AV	atrioventricular
AoV	aortic valve
AVM	arteriovenous malformation
AVR	aortic valve replacement
AVSD	atrioventricular septal defects
AVVR	atrioventricular valve regurgitation
bpm	beats per minute
BAV	bicuspid aortic valve

BT	Blalock-Taussig
ccTGA	congenitally corrected transposition of the great arteries
CHD	congenital heart disease
CI	cardiac index
CMR	cardiovascular magnetic resonance
CO	cardiac output
CoA	coarctation of the aorta
COC	combined oral contraceptive
CPB	cardiopulmonary bypass
CPEX	cardiopulmonary exercise testing
CRT	cardiac resynchronization therapy
CS	coronary sinus
CT	computed tomography
CTCA	computed tomography coronary angiography
CTR	cardiothoracic ratio
Cx	circumflex
CXR	chest X-ray
DA	descending aorta
DORV	double outlet right ventricle
DVT	deep vein thrombosis
ECG	electrocardiogram
EDP	end-diastolic pressure
EF	ejection fraction
EOL	end of life
EP	electrophysiology
ESC	European Society of Cardiology
FA	femoral artery
FBC	full blood count
Fe	iron
FU	follow-up
GA	general anaesthetic
GI	gastrointestinal
GU	genitourinary
Hct	haemocrit
HDU	high-dependency unit
HF	heart failure
HLHS	hypoplastic left heart syndrome
HR	heart rate
IART	intra-atrial reentrant tachycardia
ICD	implantable cardiac defibrillator

ICE	intracardiac echocardiography
im	intramuscular
INR	international normalized ratio
ISWT	incremental shuttle walk test
IUD	intrauterine device
iv	intravenous
IVC	inferior vena cava
IVS	interventricular septum
JVP	jugular venous pressure
L	left
LA	left atrium
LAD	left anterior descending
LAO	left anterior oblique
LAVV	left atrioventricular valve
LCAPA	left coronary artery from pulmonary artery
LFT	liver function test
LIMA	left internal mammary artery
LMS	left main stem
LPA	left pulmonary artery
LSCA	left subclavian artery
LSVC	left-sided superior vena cava
LV	left ventricle
LVH	left ventricular hypertrophy
LVOT	left ventricular outflow tract
LVOTO	left ventricular outflow tract obstruction
MAPCA	major aortopulmonary collateral arteries
MAPSE	mitral annular planar systolic excursion
mLA	mean left atrial pressure
MPA	main pulmonary artery
mPAP	mean pulmonary artery pressure
mPCWP	mean pulmonary capillary wedge pressure
MR	mitral regurgitation
mRA	mean right atrial pressure
ms	millisecond
MS	mitral stenosis
mSAP	mean systolic arterial pressure
MV	mitral valve
mVSD	muscular ventricular septal defect
NBM	nil by mouth
NICE	National Institute for Clinical Excellence

NSAID	non-steroidal anti-inflammatory drug
P-A	posterior-anterior
PA	pulmonary artery
PAH	pulmonary arterial hypertension
PAPVD	partial anomalous pulmonary venous drainage
PASP	pulmonary artery systolic pressure
PDA	patent ductus arteriosus
PFO	patent foramen ovale
PHT	pulmonary hypertension
PLE	protein-losing enteropathy
POP	progestogen-only pill
PPVI	percutaneous pulmonary valve implantation
PR	pulmonary regurgitation
PS	pulmonary stenosis
PSM	presystolic murmur
PV	pulmonary vein
PVA	pulmonary venous atrium
PVR	pulmonary vascular resistance
PVRI	pulmonary vascular resistance index
pVSD	perimembranous ventricular septal defect
QP	pulmonary blood flow
QS	systemic blood flow
R	right
RA	right atrium
RAD	right axis deviation
RAO	right anterior oblique
RAVV	right atrioventricular valve
RBBB	right bundle branch block
RCA	right coronary artery
RER	respiratory exchange ratio
RPA	right pulmonary artery
RV	right ventricle
RVH	right ventricular hypertrophy
RVOT	right ventricular outflow tract
RVOTO	right ventricular outflow tract obstruction
RV–PA	right ventricle to pulmonary artery
SC	subcutaneous
SCD	sudden cardiac death
SR	sinus rhythm
SVA	systemic venous atrium

SVC	superior vena cava
SVD	structural valve deterioration
SVR	systemic vascular resistance
SVRI	systemic vascular resistance index
TAPSE	tricuspid annular planar systolic excursion
TAPVD	total anomalous pulmonary venous drainage
TCPC	total cavopulmonary connection
TGA	transposition of the great arteries
TFT	thyroid function test
TOE	transoesophageal echocardiogram/echocardiography
ToF	tetralogy of Fallot
TPG	transpulmonary gradient
TR	tricuspid regurgitation
TTE	transthoracic echocardiogram/echocardiography
TV	tricuspid valve
U&E	urea and electrolyte
VA	ventriculoarterial
VC	valved conduit
VSD	ventricular septal defect
VT	ventricular tachycardia

Contributors

Sayqa Arif
Queen Elizabeth Hospital,
Edgbaston, Birmingham, UK

Phil Botha
Birmingham Children's Hospital
NHS Foundation Trust, UK

Sarah Bowater
Queen Elizabeth Hospital,
Edgbaston, Birmingham, UK

Paul Clift
Queen Elizabeth Hospital,
Edgbaston, Birmingham, UK

Lucy Hudsmith
Queen Elizabeth Hospital,
Edgbaston, Birmingham, UK

Nicola Pope
Queen Elizabeth Hospital,
Edgbaston, Birmingham, UK

Sara Thorne
Queen Elizabeth Hospital,
Edgbaston, Birmingham, UK

Part 1

Introduction to adult congenital heart disease

Epidemiology of ACHD

Introduction

Congenital heart disease (CHD) is the most common major congenital defect and affects approximately 1 in 100 of all newborns. Sixty years ago, only 20% of all children born with CHD survived to adulthood. This has now increased to over 90%.[1] As a result of this improved survival, there are now more adults than children with CHD in developed countries. The vast majority of these patients will require lifelong care.

Reasons for increased survival

- Improved surgical techniques.
  - Higher numbers with surgically modified disease.
- Advanced non-surgical intervention.
- Enhanced paediatric cardiac services.
- Improved diagnostic tools (e.g echocardiography, MRI).
- Prenatal diagnosis.

Due to these factors, the prevalence of complex congenital heart defects in adults has increased far more than moderate or simple defects.

Very few congenital cardiac defects are truly cured and these patients have a lifetime risk of complications including arrhythmias, heart failure, and premature death. It is therefore important that these patients are cared for by a team of professionals who understand their underlying defect, the specific type of surgical or non-surgical intervention they have undergone, and the long-term sequelae they are at risk from.

The improved survival has led to an increased age of the adult population with CHD with an increasing age at death. With advanced age they will also be at risk of developing acquired conditions such as diabetes and coronary artery disease, further contributing to their morbidity and mortality.

Cause of death in ACHD

Despite advances in care, the mortality of these patients is still higher than that of the general population. The cause of death is more likely to be cardiac in moderate and severe defects with heart failure accounting for 40% of deaths in some series.[2] There is also a higher rate of non-cardiac mortality than expected.

Cardiac causes of death include:
- Heart failure.
- Sudden cardiac death.
- Perioperative.
- Endocarditis.

1 Moons P et al. Temporal trends in survival to adulthood among patients born with congenital heart disease from 1970 to 1992 in Belgium. Circulation 2010; 122: 2264–72.

2 Nieminen HP et al. Causes of late deaths after pediatric cardiac surgery: a population-based study. JACC 2007; 50: 1263–71.

Morphology and classification

Introduction

The classification and description of complex congenital heart disease is important to the understanding of the anatomy and physiology of the conditions.[1,2] It can appear intimidating; an overview to a rational approach is described here.

1 Ho SY, Baker EJ, Rigby ML, Anderson RH. Colour atlas of congenital heart disease: morphological and clinical correlations. Times Mirror Publications Mosby-Wolfe, London; 1995.

2 Anderson RH, Becker AE. Controversies in the description of congenitally malformed hearts. Imperial College Press, London; 1997.

Physiological classification

⊃ See Table 2.1.
- A condition may be acyanotic or cyanotic.
- Acyanotic conditions may have:
  - No shunt (i.e. no communication between the pulmonary and systemic circulations).

or

  - A left (L)-to-right (R) shunt.
- Cyanotic conditions all have a R-to-L shunt.
- The behaviour of a cyanotic lesion depends on whether pulmonary blood flow is high or low (see Chapter 6, p. 61).

Table 2.1 Physiological classification of congenital heart disease

| Level of lesion | Acyanotic | | | Cyanotic—Obligatory right-to-left shunt | | | | | |
| | No shunt | Left-to-right shunt | | Eisenmenger syndrome | | High pulmonary blood flow | | Normal or low pulmonary blood flow | |
	Example of specific lesion	Level of shunt	Example of specific lesion	Level of shunt	Example of specific lesion	Level of shunt	Example of specific lesion	Level of shunt	Example of specific lesion
RV inflow	Ebstein's anomaly	Atrium	PAPVD ASD AVSD	Atrium	ASD AVSD	Atrial	Large ASD	Atrial, with obstruction to pulmonary blood flow	Severe PS with ASD, Left SVC to LA connection
LV inflow	Congenital MS, cor triatriatum	Ventricle	VSD	Ventricle	VSD	Ventricular		Ventricular, with obstruction to pulmonary blood flow	Fallot, Pulmonary atresia VSD, Univentricular heart with PS
RV outflow	Infundibular stenosis, PS	Artery	PDA AP window	Artery	PDA	Arterial		Extracardiac	Pulmonary AVM
LV outflow	Subaortic stenosis, bicuspid AoV	Multiple	AVSD	Multiple	AVSD	Multiple			
Arterial	Supravalvar stenosis, CoA								

Sequential segmental analysis

Any heart can be described using this approach. It is especially useful for complex lesions.

The heart has three segments and two junctions/connections between these segments (Fig. 2.1):
- Atrial chambers.
  - Atrioventricular connection.
- Ventricular mass.
  - Ventriculoarterial connection.
- Great arteries.

Each segment and its connection to the next is described in turn:
- Arrangement of the atria (situs)—see atrial arrangement, p. 14.
- Atrioventricular (AV) connections and the morphology of the AV valves:
  - AV concordance = normal; right atrium (RA) connects to right ventricle (RV) via a tricuspid valve (TV), left atrium (LA) connects to left ventricle (LV) via a mitral valve (MV).
  - AV discordance = abnormal; RA connects to LV via a MV; LA connects to the RV via a TV.
  - Single AV connection (one absent).
  - Double inlet AV connection.
  - Biventricular and ambiguous (isomerism).
- Ventricular mass.
  - Balanced (left and right ventricle of near equal size).
  - Unbalanced (left dominant/right dominant).
  - Solitary and indeterminate.
  - Describe relation of the ventricles to one another (topology).
- Ventriculoarterial (VA) connections and the morphology of the great arteries:
  - VA concordance = normal; RV connects to pulmonary arteries (PA) via a pulmonary valve, LV connects to aorta via an aortic valve.
  - VA discordance = abnormal; RV connects to aorta via and aortic valve, LV connects to PA via pulmonary valve.
  - Double outlet.
  - Single outlet.
- Great arteries.
  - Describe valvar and truncal relationships.
  - Trunks spiral around each other (normal) or parallel.
- Position of the heart.
  - Position: laevocardia, dextrocardia, or mesocardia.
  - Cardiac apex: points to left, middle, or right.
- Associated malformations.

The heart is considered in three segments: the atria, the ventricles and the great arteries.

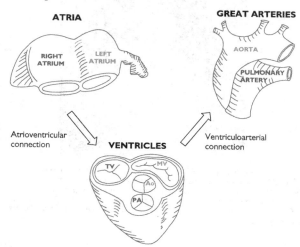

Fig. 2.1 Segments of the heart.

The heart is considered in three segments: the atria, the ventricles, and the great arteries. Reproduced from Warrell D, Cox TM, Firth JM, et al. (eds) (2003). Oxford Textbook of Medicine 4th edn, p.1084, with permission from Oxford University Press.

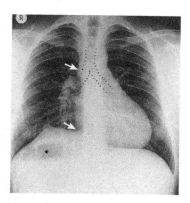

Fig. 2.2 Chest radiograph of a 50-year-old ♂ with abdominal situs inversus and laevocardia (*). Left atrial isomerism is inferred from the symmetrical long bronchi. The IVC is absent at the level of the diaphragm (small arrow) and the azygous vein receiving inferior caval venous blood is prominent (large arrow). Reproduced from Warrell D, Cox TM, Firth JM, et al. (eds) (2003). Oxford Textbook of Medicine 4th edn, p. 1084, with permission from Oxford University Press.

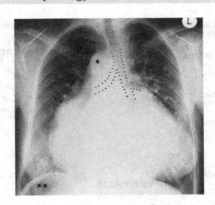

Fig. 2.3 Chest radiograph of a 21-year-old ♀ with abdominal situs inversus (**），
bronchial and inferred atrial situs inversus, mesocardia, and right aortic arch (*).
She has tetralogy of Fallot with pulmonary atresia with an aortopulmonary shunt
via a left thoracotomy. Reproduced from Warrell D, Cox TM, Firth JM, et al. (eds)
(2003). *Oxford Textbook of Medicine* 4th edn, p. 1086, with permission from Oxford
University Press.

Atrial arrangement

➔ See Table 2.2.

- Situs solitus: normal = usual arrangement of paired asymmetrical structures, i.e.
  - Morphologic left atrium (LA) on the left and right atrium (RA) on the right.
  - Morphological left main bronchus on the left and right main bronchus on the right.
  - Stomach on the left, liver on the right.
- Situs inversus = mirror image arrangement of these structures.
- Isomerism = abnormal symmetry of these structures.
  - Usually associated with coexistent complex lesions: abnormal venous connections → technical difficulties at cardiac catheterization and permanent pacemaker insertion.

Right isomerism

- More common in ♂.
- Survival to adulthood uncommon because of associated asplenia and severe cyanotic heart disease, including obstructed anomalous pulmonary venous drainage (the pulmonary venous confluence is a left atrial structure).
- Usually associated with pulmonary stenosis/atresia and often with a univentricular atrioventricular connection.

Left isomerism

- More common in ♀.
- Associated lesions tend to produce L-to-R shunts and little if any cyanosis.
- Better prognosis than right isomerism.
- In left isomerism, there is usually interruption of the inferior vena cava (IVC), and the abdominal venous return connects to the heart via a (R-sided) azygos or (L-sided) hemiazygos vein; the hepatic veins can be identified draining separately into the atria, and the posterior atrial vestibule is smooth-walled (without pectinate muscles) bilaterally.

Table 2.2 Atrial arrangement

	Atrial situs solitus: Normal	Atrial situs inversus	Right isomerism	Left isomerism
Atrial morphology	R-sided morphologic RA, L-sided morphologic LA	Mirror image: R-sided morphologic LA, L-sided morphologic RA	Bilateral morphological RA	Bilateral morphological LA
Atrial appendages	Broad-based RA appendage, long narrow LA appendage	Mirror image	Bilateral RA appendages	Bilateral LA appendages
Sinus node	Single, R-sided	Single, L-sided	Bilateral	Absent
Pulmonary morphology	R lung trilobed L lung bilobed	R lung bilobed L lung trilobed	Bilateral trilobed lungs	Bilateral bilobed lungs
Bronchial morphology*	Short R-sided main bronchus, long L- sided main bronchus	Mirror image	Bilateral short morphological R bronchi	Bilateral long morphological L bronchi
Abdominal arrangement** Aorta & IVC				
	Aorta to L of spine, IVC to R of spine	Normal or mirror image	Aorta and IVC on same side. IVC anterior to aorta	Aorta and azygos on same side; azygos posterior to aorta
Stomach Liver Spleen	L-sided R-sided R-sided	Normal or mirror image	Usually L- sided; midline usually absent	Usually R- sided; midline often polysplenia

Non-invasive imaging

Introduction

Non-invasive imaging is used extensively in patients with congenital heart disease. It is an invaluable tool in both in the initial diagnosis and also with the serial assessment and monitoring of our patients. As the technology and our knowledge continues to develop in this field, it has largely replaced the use of invasive techniques, such as cardiac catheterization, for diagnosis and assessment in many conditions.

The acquisition and interpretation of images in the different modalities of non-invasive imaging may differ significantly to that in patients with structurally normal hearts. It is important, therefore, that these tests are performed and reviewed by professionals with sufficient knowledge of the underlying anatomy and physiology, as well as the question that needs to be answered.

Chest X-ray (CXR)

This simple investigation remains an important diagnostic tool in congenital heart disease.

- Advantages:
  - Cheap, widely available.
  - Enables serial comparison.
  - Useful in emergency and acute settings.
- Disadvantages:
  - Radiation dose.
  - Structures are projected in 2D and can be superimposed.

Points to look for

- Extracardiac—bones: cervical ribs, previous thoracotomy, kyphoscoliosis.
- Prosthetic material—clips coils, prosthetic valves, devices, sternal wires (not always used post-sternotomy in children).
- Situs—gastric bubble (normally L-sided), cardiac apex (normally to the L), bronchial pattern (long L and short R main bronchus) (→ see p. 15).
- Cardiothoracic ratio (CTR).
- Cardiac silhouette —typical pattern seen with some anomalies, e.g.
  - Pulmonary atresia/Fallot —'coeur en sabot' (clog-shaped heart) (→ see Fig. 3.3).
  - Ebstein anomaly—large globular heart (measure serial CTR) (→ see Fig. 3.4).
  - Transposition of the great arteries (TGA)—'egg lying on its side' and narrow mediastinum (due to great vessels lying in an anteroposteriorly to each other) (Fig. 3.6).
- Calcification of, e.g. conduits.
- Aortic arch.
  - R-sided arch may be identified.
  - Abnormal aortic knuckle or collaterals in coarctation.
- Pulmonary arteries (PA).
  - Any dilatation of PAs.
  - Absent PAs.
- Lung vascular markings.
  - Pulmonary blood flow—plethoric or oligaemic lung fields.
  - Abnormal vascular pattern suggesting abnormal PA or pulmonary vein (PV) anatomy.
  - Dilated abnormal vessels may represent major aortopulmonary collateral arteries (MAPCAs) (→ see Pulmonary atresia with VSD, p. 156).
  - Enlarged peripheral vessels may be pulmonary arteriovenous malformations.
- Lung parenchyma—evidence of additional pulmonary disease.

Examples of the structures seen on P-A and lateral CXRs are illustrated in Figs. 3.1–3.7.

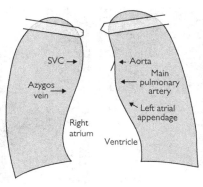

Fig. 3.1 P-A CXR—anatomical landmarks.

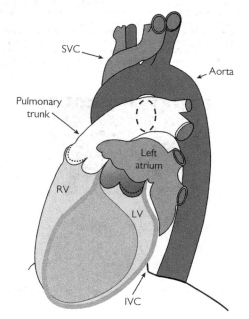

Fig. 3.2 Lateral CXR—anatomical landmarks.

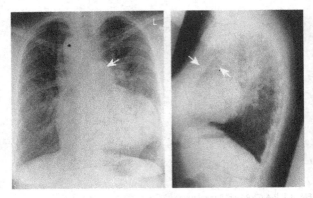

Fig. 3.3 Chest radiographs, (a) posteroanterior and (b) lateral, of a 30-year-old woman with tetralogy of Fallot and pulmonary atresia who underwent repair with a valved homograft conduit from right ventricle to pulmonary artery and ventricular septal defect closure ten years previously. There is a right aortic arch (*) and a 'coeur en sabot' cardiac silhouette. The calcification in the homograft (arrows) is more clearly seen on the lateral radiograph. The abnormal pulmonary vasculature reflects persisting aortopulmonary collaterals. Reproduced from Warrell, D et al., (2005). Oxford Textbook of Medicine 4th edn, with permission from Oxford University Press.

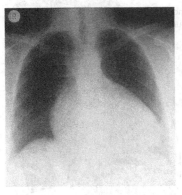

Fig. 3.4 Ebstein's anomaly with globular cardiomegaly due to dilated RA.

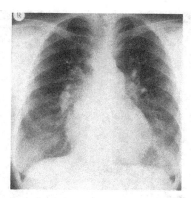

Fig. 3.5 Eisenmenger ASD—enlarged central PAs and pruning of distal vessels to give oligaemic lung fields.

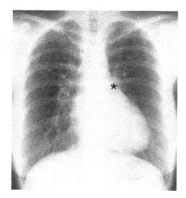

Fig. 3.6 Transposition of the great arteries. The cardiac mass has an 'egg on its side' appearance. There is a narrow mediastinum: the aorta lies directly anterior to the PA. The L heart border is straightened as the ascending aorta arises from the R ventricular outflow tract (*).

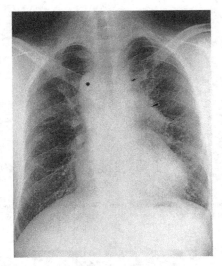

Fig. 3.7 Tetralogy of Fallot palliated with a classical left Blalock-Taussig shunt (small arrow). There is 2° dilatation of the LPA (large arrow) and a R aortic arch (*). Reproduced from Warrell D, Cox TM, Firth JM, et al. (eds) (2003). Oxford Textbook of Medicine 4th edn, p. 1091, with permission from Oxford University Press.

Transthoracic echocardiography (TTE)

- TTE is a portable and widely available imaging tool which is safe, particularly for serial imaging.
- However:
  - Experience is essential when imaging patients with congenital heart disease and studies are operator dependent.
  - Some patients, especially after surgery, may have difficult acoustic windows and there may be limited views of anterior structures.
- A sequential segmental approach should be used in all patients, especially if complex disease (➜ see Sequential segmental analysis, p. 10).
- An apical four-chamber view should be used if there are difficulties in obtaining parasternal views.
- Patients may have >1 lesion, therefore a full study should be performed.
- Basic echocardiography principles should be applied: assessment of ventricular function using dimensions and quantitative assessment including Simpson's rule, mitral annular planar systolic excursion (MAPSE), tricuspid annular planar systolic excursion (TAPSE), tissue Doppler velocities, and myocardial performance index.
- Newer techniques have improved the volumetric assessment of the patient with CHD disease using speckle tracking, strain imaging, 3D echo, and assessment of dyssynchrony.

Particular strengths of TTE

- Doppler measures of flow across valves, coarctation, shunt calculations/gradients (Fig. 3.8).
- Anatomical assessment of ventricular, atrial, and valvular structure, function (Fig. 3.9).
- Tissue Doppler assessment of ventricular function.
- Stress or exercise echo useful pre-pregnancy and for use in valvular assessment as well as ischaemia.
- Contrast echo for identification of shunts.
- Assessment of baffle leaks or obstruction.
- Identification of PVs.
- 3D assessment of valvular structure and function, particularly in repaired AVSDs, hypoplastic left heart AV valve, and Ebstein's anomaly.

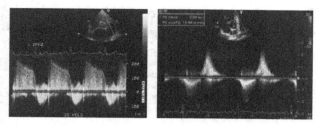

Fig. 3.8 Doppler assessment of mild (L) pulmonary regurgitation and severe (R) pulmonary regurgitation in patients with repaired tetralogy of Fallot.

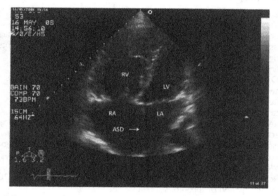

Fig. 3.9 Apical four-chamber secundum ASD with dilated RV.

Transoesophageal echo (TOE)

- Requires experienced hands for congenital heart disease patients—operator dependent.
- Care should always be taken when sedating patients: complex patients, e.g. Fontan patients, should only be sedated in expert hands and with the backup support of cardiac anaesthetists.
- Excellent views of intracardiac structures, e.g. complex outflow tracts, valve anatomy, posterior structures, e.g. abnormal or post-surgical PVs, atrial septum (see Figs. 3.10–3.13).
- Routinely used perioperatively.
- A sequential segmental approach should be followed in all patients (➔ see Sequential segmental analysis, p. 10).

Roles of TOE

- Ventricular function using 2D and 3D.
- PVs (Fig. 3.11).
- Valvular structure and function, especially the adequacy of valve repair.
- Assessment of cardiovascular connections, intracardiac repairs, shunts (Fig. 3.12).
- Periprocedural in ASD/VSD/PFO/baffle leak closure.
- 3D TOE is of significant benefit when identifying/sizing ASDs, assessing valve anatomy and function, and guiding percutaneous and surgical intervention.
- Intraoperative assessment of ventricular and valvular function, haemodynamics, adequacy of valve repairs or replacements, and surgical reconstructions.
- Assessment of intracardiac thrombus/mass and prior to cardioversion.
- Provides diagnostic information on patients with limited TTE views following previous surgery or chest deformities.
- Excellent visualization of complications of Fontan procedure (Fig. 3.10), e.g. obstruction or thrombosis.
- Visualization of atrial baffles to detect stenoses or leaks.
- Provides evaluation of AV valves and site of chordal insertion.
- Characterizes outflow tract obstructions and abnormalities of the aorta, such as CoA and PDA.
- Utilizes all techniques in acquired patients which can be translated to congenital patients in expert hands.

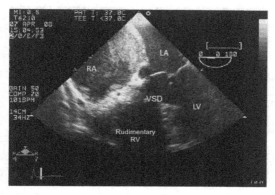

Fig. 3.10 Fontan (tricuspid atresia, TGA) with spontaneous echo contrast in the Fontan pathway (RA).

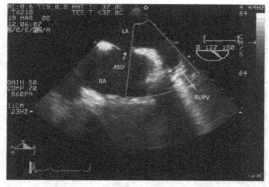

Fig. 3.11 Secundum ASD demonstrating R upper PV (RUPV).

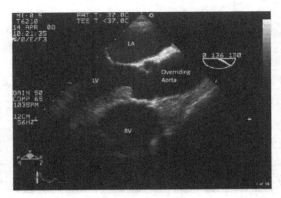

Fig. 3.12 Repaired tetralogy of Fallot demonstrating the aorta overriding the crest of the interventricular septum (*).

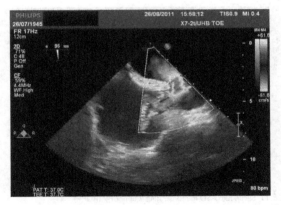

Fig. 3.13 Sinus venosus ASD with anomalous RUPV.

Cardiovascular magnetic resonance (CMR) imaging

- Gold standard method for the characterization of cardiac anatomy, function, and mass.
- Provides clear anatomical images throughout the chest.
- Accurate and reliable technique for serial monitoring of patients, particularly in response to therapeutic intervention.
- No radiation—particularly relevant to young patients with long life expectancy who require multiple scans over many years.
- Increasing availability and advancing techniques with faster acquisition.

Disadvantages, cautions, and contraindications

- Expensive.
- Requires specialist training.
- Potentially lengthy scans and breath-holds.
- Echo provides better images of fine mobile structures, e.g. valves and atrial septum.
- Some patients (2%) are claustrophobic.
- Susceptibility artefacts from stents, sternal wires, and rods from spinal deformities.
- Pacemakers, ICDs, aneurysm clips, and metallic implants are contraindicated.
  - MRI-compatible pacemakers are now available; however, the leads will still cause significant artefact within the heart.

Gadolinium contrast

- May not be needed with the advent of non-contrast MR angiography which can be acquired in <4 minutes (Fig. 3.14).
- IV gadolinium contrast can be used to provide 3D contrast angiography, assess myocardial viability, or detect the presence of scar tissue.
- Care should be used with contrast in certain patients with impaired renal function.[1]

Role of CMR in congenital heart disease

- Accurate anatomy and 'plumbing'. Beware the non-cardiac findings.
- Utilizes sequential analysis and ESC Consensus Guidelines for sequence recommendations for acquisition in congenital heart disease.[2]
- Accurate and reproducible ventricular volumes, mass, and function are essential in serial scans in young patients throughout their lifelong follow-up; e.g. repaired tetralogy of Fallot patients prior to pulmonary valve replacement (Fig. 3.15). Guidelines for the need and timing of pulmonary valve replacement utilize CMR volumes.[3]

---

1 NICE. Available at: http://www.nice.org.uk/nicemedia/pdf/CG64NICEguidance.pdf. 2007.

2 Kilner P et al. Recommendations for cardiovascular magnetic resonance in adults with congenital heart disease from the respective working groups of the ESC. Eur Heart J 2010 31(7): 794–805.

3 Geva T. Repaired tetralogy of Fallot: the roles of cardiovascular magnetic resonance in evaluating pathophysiology and for pulmonary valve replacement decision support. JCMR 2011; 13(9): doi: 10.1186/1532-429X-13-9.

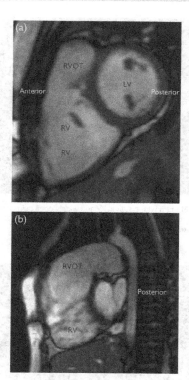

Fig. 3.14 Short-axis cardiac MR of a patient with tetralogy of Fallot showing (a) a dilated right ventricle and (b) a dilated RV patch outflow tract.

- Assessment of anatomy and function of valves acquiring regurgitant volume and fraction.
- Coarctation and aortic disease including familial aortopathies:
  - Aorta and arch/head and neck anatomy.
  - Native coarctation or recoarctation, peak velocity, and evidence of diastolic tail, collaterals (with 3D non-contrast angiography).
  - Serial assessment of aneurysms (Fig. 3.18) and dilated aorta, particularly in patients with bicuspid aortic valve (BAV).
  - Assessment of BAV anatomy and type.

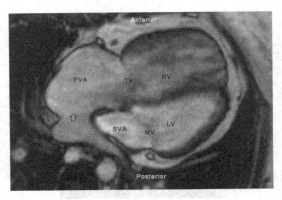

Fig. 3.15 TGA/Mustard with systemic RV and widely open pulmonary venous pathway. LV left ventricle; MV mitral valve; PVA pulmonary venous atrium; RV right ventricle; SVA systemic venous atrium; TV tricuspid valve.

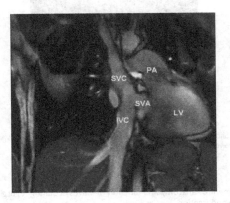

Fig. 3.16 TGA/Mustard with subpulmonary LV and widely patent systemic venous pathway. IVC inferior vena cava; LV left ventricle; PA pulmonary artery; SVA systemic venous atrium; SVC superior vena cava.

CARDIOVASCULAR MAGNETIC RESONANCE (CMR) IMAGING 35

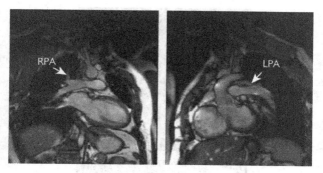

Fig. 3.17 Widely patent R and L pulmonary arteries in a repaired tetralogy of Fallot patient.

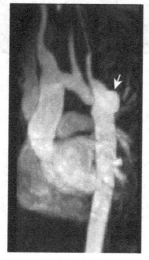

Fig. 3.18 Aneurysm formation (white arrow) at a coarctation surgical repair site.

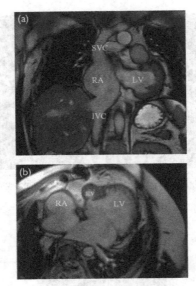

Fig. 3.19 (a) Fontan pathway with SVC and IVC entering RA and (b) dominant LV and rudimentary RV.

- Anomalous vascular branches and collaterals using 3D gadolinium contrast angiography, e.g. anomalous pulmonary venous drainage in a patient with a dilated RV.
- Assessment of shunts (e.g. PDA, ASD, VSD) by measuring the difference between pulmonary and aortic flows.
- Monitoring of operated patients: assessment of pulmonary artery stenoses (Fig 3.17), e.g. conduit patency; venous pathway patency, e.g. Mustard and Senning patients (Figs. 3.14, 3.15); tetralogy of Fallot (Fig. 3.16); Fontan connections (Fig. 3.18, 3.19); and patients with a hypoplastic left heart anatomy.

Computed tomography (CT)

- CT provides very high resolution imaging.
- Of particular use imaging coronary arteries, collateral vessels, aorta, lung, pericardial calcification.
- Improving technology and evolving applications.
- Guidelines from the Society of Cardiovascular Computed Tomography, 2015 (see Further reading).
- Advanced imaging modality of choice in patients with:
  - Contraindications to MRI, e.g. pacemakers, ICDs.
  - Prosthetic materials that cause MRI image degradation, e.g. coarctation stent, spinal rods.

Disadvantages

- The ionizing radiation dose limits repeated usage.
- Caution if using contrast in patients with impaired renal function.
- Lim,ited functional information.
- Requires sensible heart rate control (<60 bpm) for optimal image acquisition.
- Requires experienced personnel and equipment: specialist centres.

Particular uses

- Anomalous coronary arteries.
- Coronary artery disease in congenital patients.
- Assessment of RVOT patients and location/proximity of coronary arteries to potential siting of an RVOT stent/balloon.
- Coarctation stent follow-up.
- Assessment of cardiovascular connections and great vessel relations. ➔ See Fig. 3.20.
- Course of collateral vessels.
- Evidence of coronary and pericardial calcification.
- Patients with contraindications to MRI.

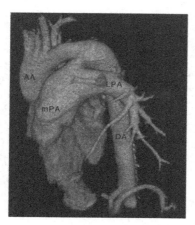

Fig. 3.20 (See also Plate 1) Eisenmenger PDA. 3D reconstruction from multislice CT scan demonstrating a PDA (arrow) in a 36-year-old woman with Eisenmenger syndrome. AA ascending aorta; DA descending aorta; LPA and mPA left and main pulmonary artery.

Further reading

Computed tomography imaging in patients with congenital heart disease: an expert consensus document. Journal of Cardiovascular Computed Tomography 2015; 9: 475–513.

Ayres NA, Miller-Hance W, Fyfe DA, et al. Indications and guidelines for performance of transesophageal echocardiography in the patient with pediatric acquired or congenital heart disease: report from the task force of the Pediatric Council of the American Society of Echocardiography. J Am Soc Echocardiogr 2005; 18(1): 91–8.

Crean A. Cardiovascular MR and CT in congenital heart disease. Heart 2007; 93: 1637–47.

Chapter 4

Physiological testing

Physiological testing

Exercise testing provides objective evidence of functional performance in cardiac disease. There are several modalities available and the method used will depend on the clinical question to be addressed, the equipment available, and the functional ability of the subject being investigated.

Indications for exercise testing

- Establishing baseline fitness.
- Determining cause of clinical deterioration.
- Determining cause of breathlessness.
- Detection of exercise-induced arrhythmia.
- Assess need for and effect of interventions.
- Work-up for heart (and lung) transplantation.
- Pre-pregnancy assessment.
- Assess suitability for competitive and leisure sports.

Testing procedures

Even for seemingly low-risk individuals, full resuscitation facilities must be available before exercise testing is performed.

Types of exercise tests

Six-minute walk test

- The six-minute walk test (6MWT) is a simple and low-tech test to perform.
- The patient is asked to walk between two cones, 30 m apart, for six minutes and is able to stop to rest as required.
- The main indication is to assess the response to medical intervention in cardiac or pulmonary disease.
- Most patients do not reach their maximal exercise capacity, thus it is a good assessment of submaximal level of functional capacity.
- This method is limited by inter-test variability.
  - Very important to standardize methods used.

Incremental shuttle walk test

- The incremental shuttle walk test (ISWT) uses a standardized protocol for patients to walk at gradually increasing speeds until they reach fatigue.
- It requires minimal equipment: just two cones and a CD.
- The patient walks between two cones, 9 m apart, with a distance around the cones of 10 m.
- A CD sounds intermittent beeps signalling the patient needs to increase their pace.
- The number of shuttles completed and total distance is recorded at the end.
- Ideally, it should be measured on two occasions due to a learning effect, with the furthest distance being recorded.
- The ISWT is highly reproducible and has been shown to be a reliable surrogate marker for peak VO_2.
- It can be used as an outcome measure to track changes in the patient's exercise capacity or to evaluate the effect of a new therapy.

Standardized Bruce exercise test

- This method is available in most hospitals.
- It allows incremental exercise with increases in both incline and speed.
- Continuous ECG monitoring is used to assess for arrhythmias and ST segment changes during exercise.
- Can be used to estimate the maximal O_2 consumption:
  - Exercise duration is measured in time expressed as decimal (T).
  - Formulae as follows, based on active and sedentary (i.e. non-athletic):
  - Male VO_2 max = 14.8 − (1.379 × T) + (0.451 × T2) − (0.012 × T3) mL/kg/min.
  - Female VO_2 max = 4.38 × T − 3.9 mL/kg/min.
- Doesn't provide evidence of maximal exercise or anaerobic threshold.

Cardiopulmonary exercise testing

- Cardiopulmonary exercise testing (CPEX), or metabolic testing, provides an objective and highly reproducible assessment of functional performance through analysis of inspired oxygen (O_2) uptake and expired carbon dioxide (CO_2) production.
- It reflects the underlying metabolic processes whilst providing an integrated assessment of cardiopulmonary function.
- This modality can assess the response to both maximal and submaximal exercise.
- It provides prognostic information in several different cardiopulmonary disease states.
- CPEX is limited by the availability of the equipment and also requires specialist knowledge for interpretation of results.

Protocol

The exercise protocol should be:
- Maximal incremental (stair-step or ramp) test.
- Ideally 8–12 min duration.

Treadmill or bicycle

- Treadmill exercise testing achieves maximal results of 10–15% higher than using a bike.
- Advantages with bicycle testing are:
  - More suitable in patients with disability.
  - Less noise when monitoring exercise blood pressure.

Measurements

Lung function

Restrictive lung defects due to previous thoracotomies or spinal abnormalities are common in congenital heart disease and therefore initial measurements of lung function are important, including:
- Forced vital capacity.
- Forced expiratory volume in 1 sec (FEV1).

Exercise testing

The patient breathes through a mouthpiece or face mask attached to a non-breathing valve. The metabolic cart directly measures inspired O_2, expired CO_2 and airflow.

Continuous ECG monitoring is performed during exercise and recovery, as well as blood pressure at defined intervals.

Frequently used terms in CPEX Reporting

- VO_2:
  - Amount of O_2 extracted from the inspired gas in a given period of time.
  - Measured in L/min or normalized to bodyweight (mL/kg/min)
- VO_2 max:
  - The highest O_2 uptake obtainable for a given exercise despite further increases in work and effort.

- VCO_2:
  - The amount of CO_2 exhaled from the body into the atmosphere per unit time.
  - Measured in L/min or normalized to bodyweight (mL/kg/min).
- VE/VCO_2 slope:
  - Assessment of ventilatory efficiency and equals the amount of air required to eliminate 1 litre of CO_2.
- Anaerobic threshold (AT):
  - The point at which aerobic respiration is supplemented by anaerobic respiration, detected by an increase in CO_2 output.
  - Measured in L/min or normalized to bodyweight (mL/kg/min).
- Minute ventilation (VE):
  - The amount of gas exhaled divided by time in minutes for gas to be collected (L/min).
- Respiratory exchange ratio (RER):
  - Ratio of CO_2 produced and O_2 consumed.
  - Surrogate marker of effort, with a peak RER <1.1 suggestive of submaximal exercise.

Reporting CPEX

The cardiopulmonary exercise report in adult congenital heart disease should contain the following information:
- Diagnosis/indication for testing.
- Exercise protocol used.
- Duration of exercise.
- Comments regarding lung function (normal/limited).
- Heart rate and blood pressure response to exercise.
- Any documented ECG changes.
- O_2 saturations.
- Metabolic gas exchange:
  - VO_2 max, AT, RER.
- Comparison with expected values and with previous tests.
- Conclusion and consequences of the test.

Data derived from the test is displayed in a Wasserman nine-panel display (see Further Reading).

Prognostic significance of results

Peak VO_2, heart rate reserve, and VE/VCO_2 slope have all been shown to be predictors of poor clinical outcomes in patients with both acquired and congenital heart disease.

Further reading

Wasserman K, Hansen JE, Sue DY, et al. Principles of exercise testing and interpretation. 4th edn. Lippincott Williams & Wilkins, Philadelphia; 2004.

Cardiac catheterization

Introduction

The purpose of cardiac catheterization in this patient group is to gain information about complex anatomy and haemodynamics, especially with respect to PA pressure and vascular resistance. In order to gain complete angiographic and haemodynamic information, studies are best performed in specialist units. In recent years, catheterization has been increasingly combined with percutaneous interventional procedures, reducing the need for further cardiac surgery in some individuals. See Table 5.1 for a list of commonly used terms and abbreviations.

Table 5.1 Glossary of commonly used abbreviations

A-P	Antero-posterior
CI	Cardiac index
CO	Cardiac output
EDP	End-diastolic pressure
FA	Femoral artery
IVC	Inferior vena cava
LAO	Left anterior oblique
LAVV	Left atrioventricular valve
LV	Left ventricle
LVOT	Left ventricular outflow tract
mLA	Mean left atrial pressure
mRA	Mean right atrial pressure
mPAP	Mean pulmonary artery pressure
mPCWP	Mean pulmonary capillary wedge pressure
mSAP	Mean systolic arterial pressure
PA	Pulmonary artery
PPVI	Percutaneous pulmonary valve implantation
PR	Pulmonary regurgitation
PV	Pulmonary vein
PVR	Pulmonary vascular resistance
PVRI	Pulmonary vascular resistance index
QP	Pulmonary blood flow
QS	Systemic blood flow
RAO	Right anterior oblique
RAVV	Right atrioventricular valve
RV	Right ventricle
RVOT	Right ventricular outflow tract
RV–PA	Right ventricle to pulmonary artery
SVC	Superior vena cava
SVR	Systemic vascular resistance
SVRI	Indexed systemic vascular resistance
TPG	Transpulmonary gradient
TOE	Transoesophageal echocardiogram
VSD	Ventricular septal defect

Indications for cardiac catheterization

Secundum atrial septal defect
- Device closure during same procedure.
- Shunt calculation and coronary angiography if unsuitable for device closure.

Coarctation (recoarctation or native)
- Measure gradient—care in passing through coarctation, consider radial approach to gain ascending aortic pressure.
- Demonstrate anatomy using contrast angiography—RAO and lateral projections (arms above head) to demonstrate coarctation.
- Consider crossing aortic valve for pullback gradient (80% bicuspid aortic valve).
- Dilation and stent deployment.

Post–tetralogy of Fallot repair
- RV function.
- Degree of PR.
- Branch PA stenosis (and dilation and stenting).
- LV function and residual ventricular septal defect (VSD).
- Coronary disease in older patient.

RV–PA conduit
- Assess conduit function—stenosis and/or regurgitation including measurement of pressure gradient through conduit.

Atrioventricular septal defect
- Look for LAVV regurgitation.
- LVOT is often elongated so care needed in measuring pullback gradient (subvalvar stenosis).
- Calculate shunt in unoperated cases.
- Coronary angiography in older patients.

Fontan
- Angiography in Fontan pathway to demonstrate pathway stenosis with follow through to look for pulmonary venous return and collaterals.
- Small pressure gradients are significant; ensure zeros are correct.
- Measure ventricular end-diastolic pressure.
- Estimate pulmonary vascular resistance.

Post–Mustard or Senning operation for TGA
- Contrast angiography for atrial pathway obstruction (and dilation and stenting).
- Atrial baffle leaks (and device occlusion).
- Systemic ventricular function and atrioventricular valve regurgitation.
- Pulmonary vascular resistance.

Precatheterization care

- Pre-hydrate all cyanotic heart disease patients with pulmonary arterial hypertension (PAH) or a Fontan circulation to reduce risk of circulatory collapse and contrast induced nephropathy.
  - 1 litre of normal saline over 12 hours whilst nil by mouth.
- Consider discontinuing warfarin two days prior to procedure and heparinize if necessary. Warfarin can be continued depending on access route, e.g. radial, brachial, jugular vein access.
- An experienced cardiac anaesthetist should be involved for all cases under general anaesthesia.
- In women of childbearing age, ensure –ve pregnancy test.
- Record height and weight.
- Shave and prep both groins (may have had previous cutdowns and multiple vascular cannulations).

Choice of catheters

Left heart catheterization

- Standard Judkins catheters are generally all that is necessary for left heart catheterization.
  - Anomalous origins of the coronary arteries are more common in congenital heart disease; therefore Williams R coronary catheter or modified Amplatz right coronary catheters may be necessary to locate the R coronary ostium.
- Ventricular angiography is best performed using a pigtail catheter. However, if following ventriculography, an accurate pullback gradient across the LVOT is necessary, exchange for an end-hole catheter such as a Judkins right 4 or MPA1. An alternative is an MPB3 which has side holes also.

Right heart catheterization

- In congenital heart disease, this requires a high level of expertise. The positioning of catheters in the right heart can be difficult due to the altered anatomy in repaired hearts, chamber dilatation, or the abnormal position of the outflow tract (e.g. congenitally corrected transposition of the great arteries (ccTGA) or post-Rastelli operation).
- For haemodynamic studies, the experienced operator will usually use a 6F MPA1 or MPB3 (Gensini) catheter as these catheters are manoeuverable; a Judkins JR4 or pigtail catheter are suitable alternatives. Care must be taken to avoid inducing arrhythmias, and pressure injections must not be given through single end-hole catheters.
- For angiography, a catheter with side holes is required, which includes the MPB3, the Pigtail, and Berman flotation catheters.
  - The advantage of the pigtail catheter is that catheter recoil is less likely during pump angiography.
  - The disadvantage of the Berman catheter is that it does not have an end hole and therefore a guide wire cannot be used to position or exchange the catheter, and a wedge trace cannot be obtained.
  - The benefit of the Berman catheter is that it is a balloon flotation catheter and it may be possible to float the catheter around a difficult subpulmonary ventricle without inducing arrhythmias.
- An alternative technique is to perform right heart catheterization via the right internal jugular vein using a Swan-Ganz catheter. This can prove to be much easier even in certain complex anatomies, including Mustard or Senning.

- Remember that if a patient is cyanotic then the balloon should not be filled with air as balloon rupture will lead to an air embolus. The balloon can be filled instead with CO_2 which will dissolve rapidly in the event of balloon rupture.
- In order to minimize the risk of catheter recoil during angiography in the PAs and subpulmonary ventricle, consider using a lower flow rate at lower pressure and with a transition time of 1 sec (e.g. 30 mL of contrast at 10 mL per sec, at 600 psi with 1 sec transition).

Routine assessments of cardiac catheterization

Always ensure zeros are correct at start of the procedure.

Oxygen saturations
- Always—IVC, SVC, PA, FA.
- If necessary—RA/RV/LV/PV.

Pressure measurements
- Right heart:
  - RA (a wave, v wave, mean).
  - RV (systolic and EDP).
  - PA (systolic, diastolic, and mean).
  - PCWP (a wave, v wave, and mean).
- Left heart:
  - FA (systolic, diastolic, mean).
  - Aortic (systolic, diastolic, mean).
  - LV (systolic, diastolic, mean).

Angiography
Ventricular angiography
- To assess function, outflow tracts, and atrioventricular valve regurgitation.
- RV (AP and lateral planes).
- LV (RAO and LAO/cranial planes).
- Interventricular septum best profiled in LV LAO/cranial view.

Aortography
- RAO 45° and LAO 45° projections.
- Assessment of:
  - Root dimensions.
  - Degree of aortic incompetence.
  - Coarctation site.
  - Aortopulmonary shunts.
  - Collateral vessels.
  - Anomalous coronary arteries.

Pulmonary arteriography
- RAO and LAO cranial planes.
- RAO projection profiles the proximal RPA.
- LAO cranial projection profiles the proximal LPA.
- Use AP cranial projection for bifurcation stenoses.

Coronary angiography
Coronary angiography should be performed if the coronary artery disease is suspected or if the patient has risk factors and is being assessed for surgery.

Coronary anomalies are common, and an initial aortogram may be useful to indicate anomalous coronary origins.

Normal values

Right and left heart
See Table 5.2.

Table 5.2. Normal values

Site	Normal range (mmHg)	Mean (mmMg)
CVP	5–8	–
RA	0–8	4
RV	15–25/0–8	EDP 5–12
PA	15–25/8–12	10–20
PCWP	9–23/1–12	6–12
Arterial/aorta	90–140/60–90	70–105
LV	90–140	EDP 5–12

Calculations

Shunt calculation by oximetry
- Mixed venous saturation = (3 × SVC + IVC) / 4.
- QP/QS = (Ao sat − mixed venous sat) / (PV sat − PA sat).

Cardiac output (CO)
- O_2 consumption (VO_2) estimated at 3 mL/kg or measured.
- Arteriovenous oxygen difference (AVO_2) = arterial − mixed venous O_2 content.
- O_2 content = sats × 1.36 × Hb.
- CO = O_2 consumption / (AVO_2 × 10) (normal 4–8 L/min).
- CO = (wt × 3) / (arterial sats − mixed venous sats) × 1.36 × Hb × 10).
- CI = CO/BSA (normal 2.5–4.2 L/min/m2).

Systemic vascular resistance (SVR)
- SVR = (mSAP − mRA) / CO (normal 10–14) Wood units.
- SVRI = (mSAP− mRA) / CI (normal 25–30).
- Multiply × 80 for SVR in dynes.sec/cm^5 (normal 700–1600) and SVRI in dynes.sec/cm^5/m^2 (normal 1970–2390).

Pulmonary vascular resistance (PVR)
- TPG = mPAP − mLAP (mPCWP).
- PVR (in Wood units) = TPG/CO (NR 1–4).
- PVRI = TPG/CI (normal 3–4).
- Multiply × 80 for PVR in dynes.sec/cm^5 (normal <250) and PVRI in dynes.sec/cm^5/m^2 (normal 255–285).

Catheter interventions in ACHD

Several catheter-based interventions can be undertaken in patients with ACHD. The aim of these is to relieve haemodynamically significant lesions, e.g. stenosis or obstruction, whilst avoiding the need for cardiac surgery. Careful pre-procedural planning, including appropriate imaging, is essential. These interventions should only be performed in specialist centres with the appropriate knowledge and expertise. These range from simple lesions, e.g. ASDs, to more complex interventions, e.g. PPVI. The majority will require long-term follow-up (FU) with serial imaging.

ASD/PFO device closure

This is covered in more detail in Chapter 9.

VSD closure

- The indications for VSD closure are mentioned in Chapter 9.
- Muscular and some perimembranous VSDs (pVSDs) are amenable to percutaneous device closure.
- Vascular access: femoral artery and right internal jugular vein.
- Periprocedural heparin (5000 units) and antibiotics given as routine.
- X-ray projections: RAO 30° + LAO 60° ± 0–20° cranial.
- Passage of catheter (MPA1, JR4, balloon-tipped catheter) from LV, through VSD into PA. Passage of wire through catheter into PA, snared and externalized via RIJ sheath, thus creating an arteriovenous circuit.
- Device placement (e.g. Amplatzer muscular VSD device) through a delivery sheath.
- pVSDs are more challenging to close percutaneously and require careful thought and expertise—significant risks of heart block which may not be apparent immediately.
- Complications: vascular haematoma, device embolization, device erosion.
- Follow-up (FU) at six weeks and annually with echocardiography plus intermittent 24-hour ECG.

PDA closure

- Closure indicated if LV volume overload or asymptomatic with audible murmur.
- Percutaneous closure treatment of choice.
- Vascular access: femoral vein and femoral artery.
- Periprocedural heparin (5000 units) and antibiotics given as routine.
- X-ray projections: AP/RAO 30° + lateral.
- Passage of catheter (e.g. MPA 1) into PA and through duct into aorta.
- Amplatz extra stiff/superstiff guidewire for support. Pigtail in aorta can be used for concomitant contrast angiography whilst deploying device.
- Commonest device: Amplatzer ductal occluder inserted through a delivery sheath.
- Device size determined by measurements on angiography.
- Complications: device embolization/erosion, vascular access site complications, risk of haemolysis with residual shunt.
- Post-procedure antiplatelet agent for six months.
- FU at six weeks and annually with echocardiography.

Aortic coarctation balloon dilatation/stent

- Indications: heart failure, hypertension, asymptomatic PG ≥20 mmHg at rest.
- In native coarctation, percutaneous insertion of stent first-choice treatment.
- Balloon angioplasty alone reserved for recoarctation in post-surgical patients ± stent placement.
- Vascular access: femoral artery ± radial artery if further contrast injections required.
- Periprocedural heparin (5000 units) and antibiotics (if stent to be inserted).
- X-ray projections: AP/slight RAO and lateral.
- Pigtail/MPB3 catheter into aorta.
- Pressure measurement and contrast angiography distal to coarctation. Stenosed segment may be easily crossed with catheter or a wire (e.g. 0.035/Terumo) may be required. Repeat pressure measurement and contrast angiography proximal to coarctation.
- Covered stents (e.g. Cheatham-Platinum covered stent) first choice— can be pre-mounted or manually mounted onto balloon (e.g. Cristal) at time of procedure.
- Stents delivered through sheath, e.g. Mullin's (sheath size 10–16 Fr).
- Need to ensure good haemostasis as often large sheath in femoral artery—manual haemostasis or use of vascular suture closure devices, e.g. Proglide.
- Stent in high-flow vessel, therefore post-procedure antiplatelet therapy not usually required.
- Complications: vascular access site bleeding/aneurysm/dissection, aortic rupture, dissection, aneurysm formation.
- FU at six weeks with CT. Annual clinical review with echo with further CT 4–5 years apart.

Pulmonary valve balloon valvuloplasty

- Indications: asymptomatic with PG >50 mmHg, right heart failure.
- First-choice treatment for congenital pulmonary stenosis.
- Vascular access: femoral vein.
- Periprocedural heparin (5000 units).
- X-ray projections: AP and lateral.
- Pigtail/MPB3 into RV—contrast angiography and passage of catheter (may need wire) through PV into PA. Lunderquist wire into distal PA for support.
- Balloon size no greater than 1.5 × diameter on echo (periprocedural TOE can be useful).
- Avoid significant PR, especially if dilated/impaired RV—can be assessed on peripocedural TOE.
- Complications—vascular complications, PR, risk of annular rupture.
- FU: 6 weeks with echo, and annually thereafter. Good long-term prognosis if no significant PR.

Aortic valve balloon valvuloplasty
- Rarely performed in adults.
- Significant risk of aortic regurgitation (AR).
- May be used as a palliative procedure in some cases.

RVOT stent
- Indications: pre-PPVI in native RVOT, palliation in native RVOT stenosis, RV–PA conduit stenosis.
- Need to ensure coronary arteries distant from RVOT—CTCA pre-procedure.
- Vascular access: femoral vein ± femoral artery (for coronary artery angiography).
- Periprocedural heparin (5000 units) and antibiotics.
- X-ray projections: AP and lateral.
- Pigtail/MPB3 in RV—contrast angiography and pressure measurements.
- Use catheter or wire to cross stenosed segment—Lunderquist wire into distal PA branch for support.
- Stent mounted onto balloon and delivered through delivery sheath.
- Simultaneous coronary angiography with balloon inflation, if concern regarding coronary artery compression.
- Complications: vascular complications, stent fracture, erosion, coronary artery compression.
- FU: 6 weeks with CXR/ECHO and annually thereafter with CXR/ECHO.

Pulmonary artery balloon angioplasty/stent
- Multiple reasons for PA/branch PA stenoses—congenital; associated with other conditions, e.g. pulmonary atresia/VSD, ToF; syndromic (Williams, Noonan); iatrogenic post-cardiac surgery (BT shunts, PA banding, ToF repair, arterial switch for TGA, pulmonary atresia/VSD repair, following Glenn procedure and arterial trunk repair).
- Indications: symptomatic; RVSP ≥50% systemic in bilateral PA stenosis or lung perfusion ≤20% in ipsilateral lung.
- Treatment options: balloon angioplasty and/or stent placement.
- Periprocedural heparin (5000 units) and antibiotics.
- X-ray projections: RPA—AP/RAO 30°; LPA—LAO°; MPA—AP cranial.
- MPA can be used to cross stenosis using 0.035 guidewire/Terumo wire. Lunderquist/Amplatz superstiff down a distal arch for support.
- Balloon/stent delivered through delivery sheath, e.g. Mullin's.
- Complications: vascular access site complications, PA trauma/rupture, aneurysm, restenosis.
- FU: 6 weeks with CXR with annual FU thereafter—serial CXR/CT.

Percutaneous pulmonary valve implantation (PPVI)

- Indications: valvular dysfunction in patients with previous surgical pulmonary valve replacement, e.g. ToF patients.
- In native pulmonary valve, RVOT pre-stenting required.
- Pre-procedural CTCA needed to ensure coronary arteries distant from pulmonary valve annulus.
- Vascular access: femoral vein ± femoral artery (for coronary artery angiography).
- Periprocedural heparin (5000 units) and antibiotics.
- X-ray projections: AP/LAO 30° cranial 20° and lateral.
- Pre-valve pressure measurements and angiography as for RVOT stenting.
- Valves in common use: Medtronic Melody valve and Edwards SAPIEN valve.
- Not suitable for people with large RVOTs.
- Complications: vascular access, infection, coronary artery compression, device embolization/erosion, valvular dysfunction, stent fracture.
- Long-term outcomes unknown.
- FU at six weeks and annually thereafter with echo.

Coil embolization

- Aortopulmonary collaterals (arise because of decreased pulmonary blood flow, e.g. pulmonary atresia; after Glenn/Fontan operations, in patients with any cyanotic congenital heart disease).
- Coronary artery fistulae.
- Venous-venous collaterals, e.g. after Glenn/Fontan surgery.
- Patients can present with haemoptysis and cyanosis.
- Closed either via coil embolization or insertion of vascular plugs.
- Pre-procedure CT aorta/arterial tree/PA may identify large collaterals.
- Detailed diagnostic angiography needed.
- Review anticoagulation if patient presents with significant haemoptysis.
- Recurrence of collaterals not uncommon.

Interventions in complex ACHD

- Fenestrations in Fontan circulations causing R → L shunts, desaturation, and risk of paradoxical emboli.
- Baffle leaks in Mustard/Senning patients due to dehiscence.
- These can be closed with Amplatzer devices.
- Baffle stenosis may require stenting if significant.
- A thorough understanding of the anatomy is essential in undertaking these procedures successfully.

Influence of pulmonary blood flow on management and outcome

Introduction

The pulmonary circulation works to transport oxygen and carbon dioxide between the airways and the cells of the body. It is able to do this whilst utilizing only very small amounts of energy itself.

The pulmonary blood flow is large, with the whole cardiac output passing through it each cardiac cycle. Despite this, pulmonary vascular resistance (PVR) is low (around 1/6 of the systemic resistance) and is able to increase and decrease through recruitment of new vessels and vascular distension. Thus, in health, the pulmonary circulation is able to accommodate a large increase in cardiac output with only a small increase in pulmonary artery pressure.

Abnormal pulmonary blood flow is frequently encountered in congenital heart disease and can have serious sequelae in both the short and the long term.

Pulmonary vascular development in early life

Fetal circulation

In the fetal circulation, the pulmonary arterial tree is muscular and non-compliant. This leads to high pulmonary vascular resistance (PVR) *in utero*. As a result of this high PVR, oxygenated blood returning from the umbilical vein is diverted into the systemic circulation, via the ductus arteriosus and foramen ovale, thus bypassing the lungs.

At birth, the newborn child starts breathing. The lungs inflate and this distension leads to dilatation of the capillary network, increased pulmonary blood flow, reduction in hypoxic-mediated vasoconstriction, and a fall in the PVR. The right atrial pressure falls and this, along with an increased left atrial pressure due to increased pulmonary venous return, leads to closure of the foramen ovale.

The elevated PO_2 in the aorta triggers contraction of the smooth vasculature in the ductus arteriosus leading to closure within the first few days of life, thus establishing the pulmonary and systemic circulations.

Normal pulmonary vascular development

- The muscular pulmonary arterial tree changes in the first few months of life:
  - The smooth muscle layer of the pulmonary arterial tree recedes from the capillary level back to the larger pulmonary arteries.
  - The pulmonary arterioles, the resistance vessels of the lungs, become non-muscular and highly compliant elastic vessels (properties that are retained throughout life).
  - These changes permit large changes in cardiac output (e.g. during exercise) without any appreciable change in PAP.
- If a child's lungs are exposed to high flow and pressure in the neonatal period (e.g. secondary to a large VSD), then these changes in pulmonary vasculature do not occur. Instead, progressive pulmonary vascular remodelling takes place, and pulmonary hypertension will develop if the defect is not repaired (Fig. 6.1).

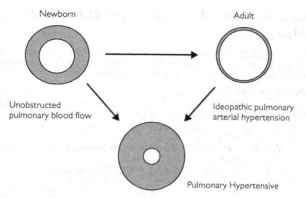

Newborn

Adult

Unobstructed
pulmonary blood flow

Ideopathic pulmonary
arterial hypertension

Pulmonary Hypertensive

Fig. 6.1 Pulmonary vascular remodelling.

Cyanotic heart disease and pulmonary blood flow

In cyanosis, there is an obligatory right-to-left shunt. That is, there is mixing of systemic and venous blood within the systemic circulation. This can be within the heart, between the great vessels, or within the lungs.

Pulmonary blood flow

In cyanosed patients, it is critical to know whether the pulmonary artery (PA) blood flow is restricted or increased.

- If the pulmonary circulation is unprotected, e.g. large VSD with no PS, the flow will be high.
  - With time, pulmonary vascular remodelling will occur and pulmonary hypertension will develop.
- If pulmonary blood flow is limited, e.g. large VSD with severe pulmonary stenosis, then pulmonary flow will be low.
  - The pulmonary arterial pressure will be low as the pulmonary vasculature is protected by the presence of the pulmonary stenosis.

Determining the pulmonary blood flow will guide intervention to either decrease (e.g. PA banding) or increase (e.g. systemic to pulmonary arterial shunt) pulmonary blood flow.

In an obligatory R-to-L shunt, normal pulmonary blood flow is indicated by systemic arterial shunts of ~85%. Higher values suggest high pulmonary blood flow, and lower values suggest insufficient pulmonary blood flow.

Pulmonary atresia

In pulmonary atresia (no blood flow into pulmonary circulation from heart), pulmonary blood flow is dependent on either:

- Collateral vessels called major aortopulmonary collateral arteries (MAPCAs) (see p. 168).

or

- Persistence of the ductus arteriosus. If the duct closes, a precipitous and perilous fall in pulmonary blood flow will occur with an associated fall in systemic saturations. The duct is therefore kept open until surgical intervention using an infusion of prostaglandin E1 (Prostin®).

Restricting pulmonary blood flow

- If the pulmonary blood flow is unobstructed, the PA is surgically banded:
  - Protects distal pulmonary circulation from high pressure flow whilst allowing adequate oxygenation.
  - The band is usually removed at later definitive surgery.
  - Adults who had a previous PA band may have mild pulmonary arterial stenosis at the site of the band.

Increasing pulmonary blood flow

If pulmonary blood flow is inadequate in early life, the patient will be cyanosed, and the pulmonary vasculature will not develop sufficiently. Pulmonary blood flow can be augmented by either a pulmonary valvotomy (either surgical or transcatheter) or using a shunt as discussed later (see Fig. 6.2).

Types of shunts to increase pulmonary blood flow

Systemic arterial to pulmonary artery shunts

- Modified Blalock-Taussig (BT) shunt—a Gore-tex® tube placed between subclavian and PAs.
- Central shunt—Gore-tex® tube between innominate and PAs.
- Classical BT shunt—subclavian to PA anastomosis (historical, no longer used).
- Waterston shunt—direct communication between ascending aorta and RPA (historical, no longer used).
- Potts anastomosis—direct communication between descending aorta and LPA (historical, no longer used).

Systemic venous-to-pulmonary artery shunt

After 4–6 months of life, the PVR has usually fallen sufficiently to allow aug-mentation of pulmonary blood supply by a systemic venous-to-pulmonary artery shunt:

- Glenn (cavo-pulmomary) shunt is a connection between the SVC and PA (see Fig. 6.3).
  - Classical Glenn: side-to-end anastomosis between SVC and RPA with RPA disconnected from MPA.
  - Bidirectional Glenn: end-to-side anastomosis between SVC and RPA. The RPA remains in continuity with main and LPA.

In children, the SVC return accounts for 70% of the total systemic venous return, thus a Glenn shunt will provide adequate oxygenation. As the child grows, the IVC accounts for a greater proportion of the venous return, and progressive cyanosis will occur. An adult with a Glenn as the sole source of pulmonary blood flow will be deeply cyanosed, as the SVC only accounts for approximately 25% of systemic venous return.

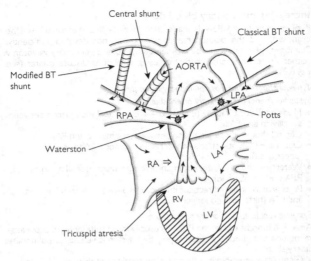

Fig. 6.2 (See also Plate 2) Types of systemic-pulmonary arterial shunts (tricuspid atresia).

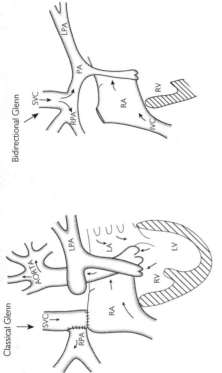

Fig. 6.3 (See also Plate 3) Systemic venous-to-pulmonary arterial shunts—the Glenn anastomosis.

Cyanosis

Introduction

Cyanosis is only present where there is a right-to-left shunt. The shunt can be at any level, e.g. intracardiac, between the great vessels, or intrapulmonary. The clinical presentation is determined by the pulmonary blood flow (see Chapter 6), and this may be low, normal, or high. Cyanosis is usually clinically detectable at SaO_2 <85%.

Due to the complexity of cyanotic congenital heart disease, it is important that all cyanotic patients are seen at a specialist centre.

Examples of cyanotic congenital defects

As before, the presentation will depend on the initial pulmonary blood flow and subsequent PVR and pulmonary artery pressure.

- Normal or low pulmonary blood flow:
  - Severe pulmonary stenosis with ASD.
  - Tetralogy of Fallot.
  - Pulmonary atresia with VSD.
  - Pulmonary arteriovenous malformation (AVM).
- High pulmonary blood flow:
  - Large VSD or AVSD.
  - Large PDA.
  - AP window.
  - Large ASD.

Defects with large left-to-right shunts that are left unoperated will develop Eisenmenger syndrome over time, with increasing PVR and a subsequent reversal of shunt direction.

Non-cardiac manifestations of cyanosis

Cyanosis is a multisystem disorder with the following widespread clinical manifestations.

- Blood and vessels (see following sections for more detail):
  - Erythrocytosis 2° to hypoxia.
  - Thrombocytopenia.
  - Coagulopathy; haemorrhage or thrombosis.
  - Fe deficiency 2° to over-venesection or menorrhagia.
  - Atherosclerotic coronary (and other systemic arterial) disease is exceedingly rare.
- Neurological:
  - Cerebrovascular accident (CVA) 2° to paradoxical embolism.
  - Cerebral abscess.
- Renal impairment:
  - Glomerular proteinuria, mesangial matrix thickening, capillary and hilar arteriole dilatation.
  - Risk of iatrogenic renal failure if dehydration occurs or with administration of nephrotoxic agents such as aminoglycosides, NSAIDs, or intravascular contrast agents.
- Gout.
- Pigment gallstones.
- Acne.
- Digital clubbing.
- Hypertrophic osteoarthropathy.

Haematological complications

Secondary erythrocytosis (polycythaemia)

Chronic hypoxaemia leads to a secondary erythrocytosis with an increased in red cell mass and haematocrit. This increases the oxygen-carrying capacity of the blood and optimizes tissue oxygenation.

The elevated haematocrit and increased blood viscosity actually correspond poorly with symptoms of hyperviscosity and are not a contributory factor to the increased risk of stroke seen in patients with cyanotic heart disease.

Venesection to reduce haematocrit

- Historically done due to concerns regarding the risks of hyperviscosity.
- Should not be done routinely.
- It does not reduce the risk of stroke.
- May cause cardiovascular collapse if simultaneous volume replacement is not given.
- May cause Fe deficiency which causes symptoms and increases the risk of stroke.
- Should only be performed for temporary relief of true symptoms of hyperviscosity (patient must be iron replete before venesection).

➔ See Table 7.1.

Table 7.1 Guidelines for venesection in cyanotic congenital heart disease

Symptoms of hyperviscosity	Haematocrit and serum Fe	Action
No	Any	Venesection not indicated
Yes	Hct >60%	Isovolumic venesection (400–500mL)
	Fe replete	
	No dehydration	
Yes	Hct <65%	Treat underlying cause of Fe deficiency
		No venesection
	Fe deficient	Consider low dose Fe therapy, closely monitoring Hct
Yes	>65%	Seek underlying cause of Fe deficiency
	Fe deficient	Avoid venesection if possible
		Consider cautious low dose
		Fe ± hydroxyurea

Coagulation abnormalities
Patients with cyanotic congenital heart disease, especially those with Eisenmenger syndrome, are at an increased risk of both bleeding and thrombosis.
- Risk of major haemorrhage:
  - Haemoptysis—especially if PAH or collaterals present.
  - During surgery.
- PA thrombosis *in situ* can occur if PHT present:
  - Associated with PA atherosclerotic changes.
  - Risk increases with age.
  - May embolize to peripheral PAs leading to hypoxia and cyanosis.
  - Anticoagulation often ineffective in resolving PA thrombus.
- Warfarin anticoagulation:
  - Use of warfarin is difficult due to risk of bleeding vs risk of thromboembolism.
  - Decision must be individualized counselling of patients with regards to risks and benefits.
  - Monitoring difficult as spuriously high INR results can occur if Hct >55 unless volume of citrate anticoagulant in sample bottle is reduced per equation below:

$$\text{Vol.citrate per mL blood} = \frac{100 - \text{Hct}}{595 - \text{Hct}}$$

Checklist for inpatients with cyanotic heart disease

- Supplemental O_2 for symptom relief only.
- Avoid iatrogenic renal dysfunction:
  - No NSAIDs.
  - Aminoglycosides only with great care.
  - IV fluids when nil by mouth (NBM) or intravascular contrast agents.
- Reduce risk of paradoxical embolism:
  - Use air filters on IV lines.
  - Use infusion pumps with bubble detector.
- Maintain adequate Hb post op for optimum O_2-carrying capacity.
- Avoid vasodilators—they increase cyanosis.
- Experienced cardiac anaesthetist for all non-cardiac surgery.
- Avoid therapies that decrease ventilatory drive:
  - Cautious use of opiates.
  - Avoid excessive O_2.

Management of common emergencies in cyanotic heart disease

Tachyarrhythmias
- Atrial arrhythmias are often atypical.
- Tachyarrhythmias are often poorly tolerated—prompt restoration of sinus rhythm required.
- DC cardioversion often safer than acute drug therapy.

Haemoptysis
- Can be life-threatening—admit.
- Urgent IV fluids, X-match blood, FFP, platelets.
- CT chest to identify site of bleeding.
- In patients with Eisenmenger syndrome, remember brachial artery BP is the same as PA pressure.
- Treat systemic hypertension with β blocker—do not use vasodilator.
- Bleeding collaterals may be possible to embolize—transfer to specialist centre.
- If major bleeding, consider selective intubation of non-bleeding lung.
- Catastrophic bleeding likely to be fatal—high-dose opiates and sedation appropriate.

Cerebral abscess
- Suspect if unexplained fever, leucoctyosis, headache, or new neurological signs.
- Urgent contrast-enhanced CT and blood cultures.
- Cerebral abscess may be presenting complaint in cyanotic disease, e.g. pulmonary AVM, anomalous systemic venous drainage.
- Cyanosis should be sought in all cases of cerebral abscess with *left-arm* bubble contrast echo to confirm.
  - right-arm injection will miss anomalously draining persistent left-sided superior vena cava (LSVC).

Part 2

Specific lesions

Valve and outflow tract lesions

Left ventricular outflow tract obstruction

Introduction

LVOTO describes a series of stenotic lesions that can occur at different levels, including:

- Subvalvar.
- Valvar—including bicuspid aortic valve.
- Supravalvar.
- Coarctation—see p. 118.

LVOTO lesions can occur in isolation or in association with other congenital cardiac anomalies. LVOTO can also occur at multiple levels, such as in Shone syndrome (see p. 87).

Irrespective of the site of the obstruction, LVOTO causes increased afterload on the LV which, if left untreated, leads to:

- LV hypertrophy.
- Eventual LV dilatation.
- LV failure.

Presentation in all types of LVOTO will depend on the severity of the obstruction and associated anomalies. It can range from an incidental murmur in mild cases to syncope or heart failure in severe obstruction. Patients with LVOTO are at risk of infective endocarditis.

Subvalvar aortic stenosis (AS)

Definition

In up to one third of patients with congenital LVOTO, the obstruction is subvalvar. There is underlying accumulation of fibroelastic tissue leading to either focal or more diffuse obstruction. In up to 90% of cases, there is a discrete or membranous subvalvar ridge (Fig. 8.1). In more severe forms there can be diffuse narrowing, leading to a fibromuscular tunnel. In rare cases, it can be caused by abnormal mitral valve tissue or chordae.

Incidence

- Prevalence of 6.5% of adults with congenital heart disease.
- Male predominance (2:1).
- Usually sporadic but familial cases reported.

Associations

- Associated with other cardiac anomalies in up to 60% of cases, including:
  - Bicuspid aortic valve.
  - Mitral valve (MV) anomalies.
  - Coarctation.
  - AVSD, VSD.
  - Shone syndrome.

Presentation

- As for other causes of LVOTO.
- Aortic regurgitation common due to functional disruption of the aortic valve.

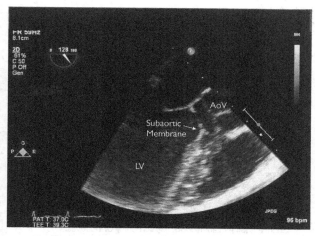

Fig. 8.1 Transoesophageal echo of a 24-year-old woman with severe subaortic stenosis due to a discrete membrane.

Natural history
- Stenosis is progressive but the rate of progression is variable.
- High rate of recurrence of obstruction despite surgical resection.

Investigation and management
- Echo delineates anatomy and severity of obstruction as well as presence of AR and associated lesions.
- Surgical repair indicated if symptomatic, or mean gradient >50 mmHg, LV dysfunction, progressive AR.
  - Surgical options include resection of membrane in discrete lesions or, if tunnel obstruction, Konno or Ross-Konno procedure.
- Long-term follow-up needed:
  - Up to 37% recurrence risk, especially in tunnel-like lesions or if resting preoperative gradient >40 mmHg.
  - Risk of progressive AR, despite surgical repair.

Bicuspid aortic valve

Definition
Bicuspid aortic valve (BAV) is due to abnormal valve development and cusp formation. As a result, there are two cusps, often of unequal size. There can be a large variation in the cusp size from nearly trileaflet to unicuspid.

Incidence
- BAV is the commonest congenital cardiac anomaly, affecting 1–2% of the population.
- Male predominance (4:1).
- Both sporadic and inherited forms:
  - Autosomal dominant with variable penetrance.
  - First-degree relatives of patients with any type of LVOTO are at a higher risk of BAV.

Associations
- Aortopathy of the ascending aorta:
  - Similar to Marfan syndrome with medial disease.
  - Aortic root dilatation.
  - Risk of dissection.
- 20% have other anomalies, e.g. coarctation, patent arterial duct.

Presentation
- Depends on severity of obstruction, including:
  - Severe *in utero* aortic stenosis (AS) leading to failure of the left ventricle to develop (hypoplastic heart syndrome—p. 174).
  - Severe AS requiring surgical repair in infancy.
  - Chance finding in adulthood, e.g. screening of relatives.
- AS is the most common sequela, but aortic regurgitation (AR) can also occur.
- Usually progressive, especially if cusps are very unequal in size or if unicuspid.
- Probability aortic valve replacement (AVR) increases from 1% at 1–9 years to 30% at 60–69 years.
- Aortic root dilatation can occur even in the absence of AS or AR:
  - Not stopped or reversed by AVR.

Investigation and management
- Symptoms occur late in young people, so regular follow-up important.
- CXR—dilatation of ascending aorta (AA).
- ECG—LVH and left axis deviation if severe AS.
- Echo to monitor AV function, LV dimensions and function, associated anomalies.
- Exercise testing (medically supervised) in moderate-to-severe asymptomatic AS—intervene if ST segment changes, failure of BP to rise.
- Serial MRI if aortic root dilation.

Intervention
Intervention should be considered if:
- AS:
  - Symptoms or LV dysfunction and severe AS (mean gradient >50 mmHg).
  - Asymptomatic severe AS with abnormal exercise response.
  - Less severe but coexistent lesion such as moderate or severe AR or dilated aortic root.

- AR:
  - Symptoms and moderate-to-severe AR.
  - Asymptomatic severe AR if progressive LV dilation or LV impairment.
- Balloon valvuloplasty can be used, especially in children or young adults when the leaflets are still pliable with minimal calcification.
- In most adult cases, aortic valve replacement (AVR) is the treatment of choice.
- Choice of valve depends on lifestyle, plans for pregnancy, and coexisting lesions:
  - Prosthetic AVR.
  - Tissue AVR.
  - Ross procedure—pulmonary autograft.

Supravalvar AS
Definition
Supravalvar AS is the rarest type of LVOTO. The lesion can be either focal or more diffuse narrowing, starting at the sinotubular junction and can involve the entire ascending aorta.

It is most commonly associated with Williams syndrome, but a rare sporadic form and an autosomal dominant form can also occur. In all three types, there is a mutation of the elastin gene on chromosome 7q11.23.

Associations
- Williams syndrome (elfin-like face, short stature, low IQ).
  - May also have stenosis of any artery including PAs, renal arteries, and descending aorta.
- Aortic valve abnormalities found in up to 50%, most commonly bicuspid valve.

Natural history and presentation
- Patients will typically present with other features of Williams syndrome.
- Other patients present similar to other forms of LVOTO.
- Patients with supravalvar AS may present with myocardial ischaemia due to:
  - Fibromuscular thickening that may encroach into the coronary ostia.
  - The coronary arteries are proximal to the obstruction, so the coronary circulation is exposed to high LV pressures.
  - Coronary involvement is associated with a worse prognosis than other forms of LVOTO.

Investigation and management
- Echo—anatomy and severity of supravalvar stenosis.
- MRI/CT—assess involvement of whole aorta and pulmonary tree.
- Cardiac catheter—assess severity of stenoses and coronary involvement.
- Surgical repair should be considered if:
  - Symptoms.
  - Coronary involvement.
  - Mean pressure gradient >50 mmHg.

Left ventricular inflow lesions

Congenital mitral valve abnormalities

Congenital abnormalities of the mitral valve (MV) are very rare and most commonly give rise to obstructive defects. They are usually found in association with other cardiac defects such as LVOTO, coarctation, ASD, VSD, or tetralogy of Fallot.

Types

Supra-mitral ring
- A membrane is present in the left atrium immediately above the mitral valve and inferior to the appendage.
  - This differs to cor triatriatum in which membrane is superior to appendage.
- Membrane causes obstruction of the MV and may also restrict leaflet motion.

Parachute mitral valve
- Single, abnormal papillary muscle into which all chordae tendineae insert.
- Both the valve and subvalvar apparatus are often dysplastic.
- Obstruction occurs at the level of the papillary muscles.

Mitral arcade
- Chordae tendineae are either absent or shortened.
- The leaflets are thickened and insert directly into papillary muscle.
- Excursion of the leaflets is restricted and results in mitral stenosis (MS).

Double orifice mitral valve
- A fibrous bridge of excess leaflet tissue partially or completely divides the mitral valve orifice.
- MS can occur due to restricted excursion of mitral leaflets.
- Valve may also be regurgitant.

Presentation
- Majority of these defects are diagnosed and repaired in childhood.
- Those detected in adulthood are usually mild and often present due to associated defects.
- Unoperated cases reaching adulthood are usually mild and may present due to associated defects.

Investigation and management
- Echocardiography defines the anatomy, degree of obstruction, and associated defects.
  - Severity of MS may be underestimated if coexistent ASD.
  - L-to-R shunt in coexistent ASD will be increased by significant MS.
- Surgical repair indicated if significant obstruction.

Cor triatriatum

- Cor triatriatum is a rare defect most commonly affecting the left atrium but may affect the right atrium too.
- A fibromuscular membrane, perforated by ≥1 holes, divides the atrium into two chambers:
  - Upper accessory chamber receives pulmonary venous return.
  - Lower chamber is the true LA with appendage and MV.
- Associated cardiac defects occur in 70–80% (ASD in 50%).

Presentation

- The presentation will depend on the communication between the two chambers.
- If the hole(s) in the membrane are restrictive, pulmonary venous obstruction and supravalvar mitral stenosis will occur and the patient will usually present in childhood.
- If little or no obstruction, the patient may present in adulthood with:
  - Incidental finding requiring no treatment.
  - Increasing pulmonary pressures.
  - Atrial fibrillation.
  - Development of mitral regurgitation.

Investigation and management

- CXR:
  - Pulmonary congestion.
- TOE:
  - Anatomy, functional significance, associated lesions.
  - L atrial appendage not dilated because in low pressure lower chamber.
- Surgical resection of membrane indicated if causing obstruction to pulmonary venous flow.

Shone syndrome

Shone syndrome, or complex, is a series of lesions causing obstruction to left ventricular inflow and outflow. In its complete form there is:
- Supra-mitral ring.
- Parachute MV.
- Subvalvar AS.
- Coarctation.

Presentation

- The presentation and prognosis will depend on the degree of obstruction and its effect on blood flow.
- The majority of patients will present in childhood.

Investigation and management

- Transthoracic echo, TOE, and MRI will assess for the presence of all four lesions and the degree of obstruction.
- Surgical repair of significant coarctation is usually performed in neonatal period.
- Patients may require multiple operations to relieve the different levels of obstruction.

Right ventricular outflow tract obstruction (RVOTO)

Introduction
RVOTO can be due to narrowing at one or more of the following levels:
- Mid–right ventricle (RV).
- Infundibulum.
- Pulmonary valve.
- Supravalvar region.
- Branch or peripheral pulmonary arteries (PA).

Whilst most cases of RVOTO are due to underlying congenital lesions, it can also arise from prior surgery, such as a previous Blalock-Taussig shunt or conduit stenosis.

RVOTO results in elevated right ventricular pressure and if sustained, RV hypertrophy will develop. This can remain asymptomatic for many years before the development of RV dilatation or reduced cardiac output.

Pulmonary valvar stenosis
Pulmonary stenosis (PS) is the commonest type of RVOTO, occurring in up to 10% of patients with congenital heart disease. It is usually found in isolation but can be associated with other defects, including ASDs or peripheral PA stenosis.
- There are two main morphological types:
  - Thin, pliable leaflets with dome shape (80–90% cases); often associated with a dilated PA.
  - Dysplastic valve with thickened and immobile leaflets; the RVOT and annulus are often narrowed.
- Valvar PS can also be associated with several syndromes, including:
  - Noonan syndrome.
  - Williams syndrome.
  - Alagille syndrome.
  - Congenital rubella syndrome.

Symptoms
- Rare in mild-to-moderate stenosis.
- Severe stenosis may present with:
  - Decreased exercise tolerance.
  - Dyspnoea.
  - Chest pain.
  - Atrial arrhythmias.

Physical signs
Key features include:
- May have phenotypical appearance if associated with a syndrome.
- RV heave if right ventricular hypertrophy (RVH) present.
- Prominent 'a' wave in jugular venous pressure (JVP) due to forceful RA pressure.
- Soft delayed P2.
- Ejection systolic murmur at L upper sternal edge—increases with inspiration.

- Systolic ejection click if the leaflets are thin and pliable.
- Cyanosis if severe PS + coexistent PFO or ASD.

Natural and operated history
- Mild PS (PG <30 mmHg) rarely deteriorates.
  - May not need long-term follow-up once adulthood reached.
- Moderate PS may progress and need intervention in ~20% cases.
- After balloon or surgical valvuloplasty, pulmonary regurgitation is common which may, in time, result in RV dilatation and eventual failure; thus all require lifelong follow-up post-intervention.

Investigations
Key points to look for:
- ECG—severe PS: p pulmonale, R axis deviation (RAD), R ventricular hypertrophy (RVH).
- CXR—dilation of main PA, decreased pulmonary vascular markings.
  - Chen's sign = vascular fullness at L base due to preferential flow of turbulent jet into LPA.
- Echo—PV anatomy and severity of PS, RV size and function, associated cardiac abnormalities.
- MRI—quantify RV size and function, identify any branch or peripheral pulmonary arterial stenoses.

Intervention
Intervention should be considered if PS is severe (peak pressure gradient >50 mmHg) or if symptoms or RV dysfunction present.

Percutaneous intervention
- Balloon valvuloplasty:
  - Similar long-term results to surgical repair.
  - Suitable for dome-type stenosis when leaflets are pliable.
- Percutaneous valve replacement—new technique, suitable for selected cases, available in limited number of centres.

Surgical intervention
- Valvotomy—subsequent PR more frequent than post-percutaneous intervention.
- Valve replacement.

Supravalvar pulmonary stenosis
- Rarest form of PS.
- Caused by ring of hypertrophic tissue at the sinotubular junction of main PA.
- Associated with congenital rubella and Williams syndrome.
  - Obstruction may occur at multiple levels throughout the pulmonary vasculature.
- Iatrogenic supravalvular PS may occur post-surgery involving main PA (Fallot, arterial switch, and PA banding).
- Examination findings are identical to valvar PS, except the absence of a click (suggests normal pulmonary valve).
- Balloon dilatation is rarely successful, and surgical correction is usually required if severe.

Pulmonary artery stenosis
- Branch PA stenosis most commonly affects main and lobar arteries.
- Associated with Williams and Alagille syndromes.
- Iatrogenic PA stenosis may occur following systemic to PA shunts or arterial switch operations.
- Isolated PA stenosis rare.
- First-line treatment is balloon dilatation ± stent.
  - Caution required in post-arterial switch patients due to the close relation of the PAs straddling either side of the aorta.

Pulmonary atresia with intact septum
- Very rare.
- There is complete RVOTO with varying degrees of RV and TV hypoplasia and an intact intraventricular septum.
- PAs are usually small but have normal branching pattern.
- Untreated, this is universally fatal.
- Neonatal management includes systemic-pulmonary arterial shunt (Blalock-Taussig) ± surgical or transcatheter procedure on the RVOT to augment PBF.
- Subsequent management will depend on the size of the RV and its ability to support the pulmonary circulation:
  - If RV is small, biventricular repair is unlikely, and the patient will be considered for a Fontan operation.

Double-chambered right ventricle
- Anomalous muscle bundles divide the RV into two chambers:
  - High pressure proximal chamber.
  - Low pressure distal chamber.
- VSD present in 75% cases—usually distal to the level of obstruction.
- Other associations include:
  - Valvar PS.
  - Tetralogy of Fallot.
  - Double outlet RV.
  - Subaortic obstruction.
- Obstruction may be mild in childhood but progresses in adulthood as progressive RVH develops.
- Cyanosis may develop if coexistent PFO/ASD or if VSD is proximal to level of obstruction.
- MRI is the best imaging modality to assess level of obstruction.
- Treatment is surgical resection of obstructing muscle bands and closure of VSD if present.

Ebstein anomaly

Definition

Ebstein anomaly arises when there is a failure of delamination of the septal and posterior leaflets of the tricuspid valve (TV). These leaflets are adherent to the myocardium and are often thickened and hypoplastic. The anterosuperior leaflet is large but tethered and is often fenestrated. It may be displaced into the RVOT.

As a result of these changes, the functional annulus is displaced into the RV cavity, away from the atrioventricular ring. This leads to:
- Atrialization of the proximal part of the RV → enlarged RA.
- Small functional RV.
- Tricuspid regurgitation (TR).

➔ See Fig. 8.2.

Incidence
- Rare—approximately 1 in 20,000 live births, 0.5% of all congenital heart disease.
- Equal sex incidence.
- Majority of cases are sporadic.
- Associated with maternal ingestion of lithium in the first trimester.

Associations
- ASD or PFO in majority of cases.
- 25% Wolf-Parkinson-White syndrome, often with multiple pathways.
- May form part of other complex lesions—tetralogy of Fallot, VSD, PDA, and congenitally corrected TGA.
- High incidence of left heart anomalies, including abnormalities of the LV, such as non-compaction.

Natural history
This can be extremely variable and ranges from intrauterine death to presentation in late adulthood. The age at presentation depends on:
- Degree of leaflet displacement.
- Amount of tricuspid regurgitation (TR).
- Functional capacity of RV.
- Associated lesions.

Presenting features in the adult
This will again depend on the severity of the tricuspid regurgitation, the RV function, and the degree of right-to-left shunting across the interatrial septum. Presenting features include:
- Murmur.
- Arrhythmia.
- Features of right-sided heart failure.
- Progressive cyanosis.
- Paradoxical embolism.

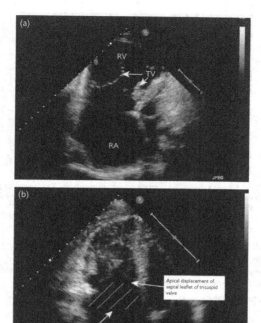

Fig. 8.2 (a) and (b) Ebstein anomaly transthoracic echocardiography. Apical four-chamber views showing tricuspid valve displacement towards the R ventricular apex. The functional RA is very dilated, due to atrialization of part of the RV.

Physical signs

- Cyanosis and clubbing (if R-to-L shunt through ASD or PFO).
- Elevated JVP is a late sign because the TR regurgitant volume is accommodated by the large capacity functional RA.
- Widely split S1 due to increased excursion of anterosuperior leaflet.
- Widely split S2 due to delayed P2 (RBBB).
- Tricuspid regurgitant murmur varies from very soft to loud enough to generate thrill.
- Signs of RV failure are late and include hepatomegaly, ascites, and peripheral oedema.

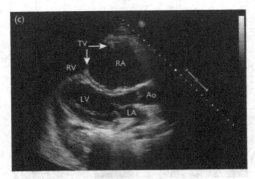

Fig. 8.2 (c) Ebstein anomaly—transthoracic echocardiography. Parasternal long axis view, showing compression of the LV by the dilated right heart. Ao aorta; LA left atrium; LV left ventricle; RA right atrium; RV right ventricle; TV tricuspid valve.

Investigations

Chest X-ray
- Characteristic silhouette and cardiomegaly due to RA enlargement; small aortic knuckle and oligaemic lung fields.

Electrocardiography
- Superior axis.
- First-degree heart block (50%).
- RBBB.
- Low-voltage QRS complexes over right chest leads.
- Pre-excitation (25%).

Echocardiography
- Confirms diagnosis—apical displacement of septal ± posterior TV leaflet of >8 mm/m^2.
- Key to planning surgical repair:
  - Anatomy and function of TV.
  - RV size and function.
  - Size of functional RA.
  - Associated structural defects.

MRI
- Assessment of RV volumes and function.

Cardiopulmonary exercise test
- Detection of early limitation due to a deterioration in cardiac function.

Management

Non-surgical options

- Symptomatic treatment of heart failure.
- Anticoagulation if atrial arrhythmia present.
- Ablation of accessory pathways.
- Higher rate of recurrence than for structurally normal hearts.
- Device closure of PFO/ASD if cyanosis and only mild-to-moderate TR.
  - TR may worsen with closure of ASD, so must be assessed carefully.

Surgical options

Surgery to repair or replace the TV should be performed before the RV started to fail. It should be considered if:

- Increasing RV volumes/decreasing RV function.
- Reduction in objective exercise tolerance or functional capacity.
- Significant arrhythmias.

Successful repair of the TV is technically difficult and therefore surgery should be carried out only in selected tertiary centres. Surgical options include:

- TV replacement.
- TV repair—preferable to replacement with lower mortality and long-term complications.
- Plication of atrialized RV.
- Right atrial MAZE procedure.
- Closure of ASD/PFO.
- If RV function is poor, a 1.5 ventricle repair can be considered with cavopulmonary shunt to reduce pre-load to the RV.
- Cardiac transplantation if severe biventricular failure.

Septal defects

Atrial septal defects

Introduction
The true atrial septum lies within the rim of the oval fossa whilst the rest of the wall that separates the left and right atrium is actually made of infolds of tissue arising in early fetal development. However, all defects that lead to shunting at an atrial level are usually referred to as atrial septal defects. The different types of atrial septal defect (ASD) are illustrated in Fig. 9.1.

In normal circumstances, ASDs will shunt left to right. The size of this shunt is determined by the size of the defect, the right ventricular compliance, and the pulmonary vascular resistance.

The different types of ASDs account for ~10% of congenital heart disease.

Ostium secundum ASD

Definition and incidence
- Ostium secundum ASDs describe defects of the oval fossa (i.e. the true atrial septum) which allow shunting of blood at an atrial level.
- Common anomaly accounting for 60% of all ASDs.
- ♀:♂—2:1.

Associations
- Cardiac associations include:
  - MV disease—stenosis (MS + ASD known as Lutembacher syndrome), prolapse, or regurgitation.
  - Pulmonary vein stenosis.
  - VSD.
  - PDA.
  - CoA.
  - Tetralogy of Fallot.
  - Partial anomalous pulmonary venous connection.

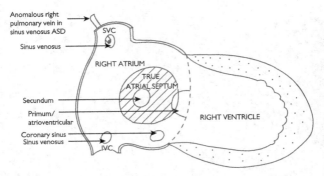

Fig. 9.1 Sites of ASDs. The shaded area delineates the true atrial septum. Sinus venosus and coronary sinus defects are therefore not strictly ASDs although they permit shunting at atrial level.

- Genetic syndromes:
  - Can be familial with autosomal dominant inheritance, associated with delayed AV conduction.
  - Down syndrome.
  - Holt-Oram syndrome—autosomal dominant condition with skeletal abnormalities and AV conduction defects, due to *TBX5* mutation.

Presentation
- Childhood:
  - Isolated ASDs are usually asymptomatic and may present with a murmur.
  - May present with dyspnoea or recurrent chest infections; sometimes misdiagnosed as asthma.
- Adulthood:
  - Can remain undiagnosed for years if symptoms are mild, due to the signs being subtle and easily missed.
  - Most commonly present with progressive exertional dyspnoea and palpitations.
  - May be diagnosed after cardiomegaly found on a CXR or CT thorax.

Natural history if unrepaired
- Complications of an ASD with a significant shunt include:
  - Atrial fibrillation/flutter—20% by 40 years.
  - Right heart failure.
  - Mitral/tricuspid regurgitation.
  - LV dysfunction.
  - PAH: mild PAH (<6 Wood units) is common with advancing age. Only 10% of ASDs develop severe PAH with a R-to-L shunt. The pulmonary vascular bed is not exposed to systemic pressures in ASDs, and the causal relationship between ASD and Eisenmenger syndrome remains controversial.
  - Systemic arterial hypertension.
  - Paradoxical embolism.
  - Endocarditis.
- Elevated LA pressure will increase the L-to-R shunt and increase symptoms.
  - LV dysfunction with increased LVEDP.
  - MV disease—LA pressure increased in both MS and MR.

The severity of MS and MR is underestimated when an ASD coexists, as the LA can decompress through the ASD. If significant MS or MR is missed and the ASD closed, patient may decompensate dramatically.

Physical signs
Points to look for:
- Loud S1, widely split and fixed S2.
- Pulmonary ejection systolic murmur at upper L sternal edge.
- Tricuspid mid-diastolic murmur at lower L sternal edge (due to ↑ flow across TV).

- If R heart failure or PAH:
  - Raised JVP.
  - RV heave at L sternal border.
  - Palpable PA in L second intercostal space.

Investigation

Points to look for:
- ECG—sinus node dysfunction, prolonged P-R interval, RAD, rSr pattern in V1, large P waves.
- CXR—dilated proximal PAs, small aortic knuckle, plethoric lung fields, cardiomegaly (dilatation of RA and RV).
- TTE—dilated, volume overloaded RV, colour flow across interatrial septum, Doppler estimate of PA pressure and any associated lesions.
- Transoesophageal echocardiogram—define number, site, size, and margins of ASD; identify PVs.
- Cardiac catheterization—calculation of pulmonary vascular resistance and assessment of coexistent congenital or acquired cardiac pathology, e.g. coronary artery disease.

ASD repair

Indications for closure of ASD
- R heart volume overload.
- L-to-R shunt ≥1.5:1 and ASD ≥10 mm in diameter.
- Prevention of recurrent paradoxical embolism.
- Benefits of closure of haemodynamically significant ASD are improved:
  - Survival.
  - Functional class.
  - Exercise tolerance.
  - Reduction of risk of heart failure.

Contraindications to ASD closure
- Significant pulmonary vascular disease.
- Severe LV dysfunction.
- Significant MV disease.

Percutaneous device closure of ASD
- Percutaneous closure may be performed for isolated secundum ASD if:
  - <4 cm diameter.
  - Anatomically away from AV valves, pulmonary and caval veins.
  - Normal pulmonary venous drainage.
  - Pre-procedure TOE essential to anatomy is suitable—size and adequate rims (≥5 mm).
- Performed either under GA with TOE guidance or using conscious sedation with intracardiac echocardiography (ICE).
- Vascular access: femoral vein (initially 6F sheath).
- Periprocedural intravenous heparin 5000 units and antibiotics.
- Working view: AP or LAO 30°.
- MPA1 catheter to measure PA pressure.
- Cross ASD with MPA1 catheter ±0.035˝ guidewire and advance into a pulmonary vein.
- Amplatzer superstiff 180 cm wire into PV for support.

- Devices: Amplatzer atrial septal occluder, Gore septal occluder, Cera septal occluder, Occlutech Figulla occluder, and Biostar (biodegradable device).
- Devices delivered through a delivery sheath.
- Use fluoroscopy and echocardiography to deploy device.
- Risk—1–2% major complication: vascular complications, death, stroke, device embolization/erosion.
- Antiplatelet therapy recommended for six months post-closure.
- Follow-up: six weeks with echo, with annual surveillance thereafter.
- Some reports of late erosion.

The alternative to percutaneous closure is surgical repair ± MAZE procedure. Mortality similar to device closure, but there is a higher incidence of post-operative AF and recovery is longer.

Prognosis post–ASD repair
- Repair by 20 years—normal life expectancy, late complications unlikely.
- Repair after 25 years—late atrial arrhythmia may occur.
- Repair after 40 years—functional capacity improved, longevity may be less than normal population but better than if unrepaired.

Ostium primum ASD
Definition
An ostium primum defect is a defect of the true atrial septum and may also be described as an endocardial cushion defect (➔ see Fig. 9.1, p. 95). It is usually seen as part of an atrioventricular septal defect and is discussed later (p. 108).

Sinus venosus ASD
Definition and incidence
- Sinus venosus defects are not true ASDs but permit shunting at an atrial level.
- They are due to defects of the infolding of the atrial wall at the site of the SVC or IVC.
- Superior sinus venosus defects are more common than the inferior defects.
    - The defect of the atrial wall leads to the SVC communicating with both atria.
    - Usually associated with anomalous right-sided pulmonary veins which drain into the SVC near its junction with the atria.
- Sinus venosus defects account for 2–3% of ASDs.
- Equal sex incidence.

Associations
- Anomalous pulmonary venous drainage.
- Ectopic atrial pacemaker (defect in area of SA node)—look for leftward p wave axis and inverted p wave in lead III.

Presentation
As for secundum ASD.

Diagnosis
- TOE required to visualize defect and associated anomalous pulmonary venous drainage.
- MRI and CT can be used to identify PAPVD if not seen clearly on TOE.

Management
- The indications for closure are the same as for secundum ASDs.
- Sinus venosus defects are not suitable for percutaneous drainage as deficient superior rim and anomalous venous drainage often present.

Coronary sinus defect
- This is the rarest of all ASDs and is due to a defect of the entry site of the coronary sinus to the left atrium.
- In its mildest form, there is a simple fenestration in the atrial wall by the opening of the coronary sinus.
- Unroofed coronary sinus is a variation of this defect in which the roof separating the coronary sinus from the LA is absent.
  - A persistent LSVC draining to the coronary sinus usually coexists, resulting in a R-to-L shunt and cyanosis.
- Presentation is as for secundum ASD but also cyanosis.
- TOE ± cardiac catheterization needed for further assessment.
- Management is with surgical repair.

Patent foramen ovale (PFO)
Definition and incidence
- PFO is a normal variant found in up to 25% of the population and does not constitute a congenital cardiac defect.
- Results from failure of fusion of the valve of the foramen ovale with the septum after birth when the LA pressure exceeds that of the RA—there is no deficiency of atrial septal tissue.

Presentation
- Incidental finding.
- Paradoxical embolism or embolism of thrombus *in situ*:
  - Cryptogenic stroke in young adults.
  - Neurological decompression sickness following diving.
- Migraine with aura may be associated with PFO.

Physical signs and investigations
- Signs—none, except from any previous neurological deficit.
- ECG, CXR, and TTE are normal.
- Contrast echo:
  - PFO is likely if, with Valsalva, bubbles appear in the LA within five heartbeats.
  - Should only be performed if there is a plan to close the PFO—knowledge of the existence of a PFO for which there is no indication for closure may cause unnecessary anxiety.

Indications for closure of PFO

- Patients with previous embolic stroke, PFO, and risk factors for venous thrombosis appear to be protected against further events by device closure.
- Careful risk assessment must be made in all patients with an embolic stroke prior to device closure because if multiple risk factors (e.g. smoking, hypertension, diabetes, hyperlipidaemia, or proven atherosclerotic disease) or factors for L-sided intracardiac thrombosis (e.g. AF, MV disease with a dilated LA) are present, device closure is unlikely to reduce further events.
- Other indications for closure include decompression illness and platypnoea-orthodeoxia.
- There is no proven benefit for PFO closure in migraine sufferers.
- Percutaneous closure is performed as for secundum ASDs. Antiplatelet therapy is recommended for six months post-procedure. However, a single antiplatelet agent should be continued long term if arterial thromboembolism was a possible cause for the neurological event.

Ventricular septal defects (VSDs)

Definition and incidence

- The interventricular septum is made up of four parts: inlet septum, outlet septum, muscular septum, and perimembranous septum (see Fig. 9.2).
- VSDs can arise from defects in any of these components and are classified by their location within the septum and by their borders as viewed from the RV:
  - Muscular VSD.
  - Perimembranous VSD (pVSD).
  - Doubly committed subarterial VSD.
- Commonest type of congenital heart defect affecting 3/1000 live births.
  - pVSD is the commonest type of VSD found in Europe and North America.
  - Doubly committed VSDs account for 30% of VSDs in Asian population compared to 5% in European and North American populations.
- Equal sex incidence.

Cardiac associations

Occurs as:
- Isolated defect.
- In association with other lesions, e.g. coarctation.
- As integral part of more complex condition, such as tetralogy of Fallot.

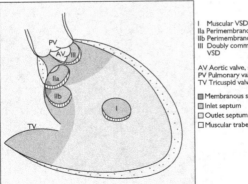

I   Muscular VSD
IIa Perimembranous outlet VSD
IIb Perimembranous inlet VSD
III Doubly committed subarterial VSD

AV Aortic valve, seen through VSD
PV Pulmonary valve
TV Tricuspid valve

▨ Membranous septum
▨ Inlet septum
▢ Outlet septum
▢ Muscular trabecular septum

Fig. 9.2 (See also Plate 4) Schematic representation to show the sites of different types of VSDs. The heart is in cross-section, viewed from the R ventricular aspect.

Presentation

The mode of presentation will depend on the size and haemodynamic effects of the VSD.
- Restrictive VSDs describes small defects with a large pressure gradient between the left and right ventricles and a small shunt of no haemodynamic significance.
- Moderate size defects (Qp:Qs 1.5–2.5:1) are haemodynamically significant and will cause volume overloading of the left ventricle.
- Large defects (Qp:Qs >2.5:1) present early in life with left ventricular overload and progressive pulmonary vascular disease (unless coexistent RVOTO).

Children
- Small defects are often asymptomatic, but loud systolic murmur. Spontaneous closure of perimembranous or small muscular VSD is common.
- Moderate or large VSDs will present with failure to thrive and congestive heart failure.

Adults
- Unoperated restrictive VSDs usually asymptomatic.
- Survivors of large unoperated VSDs are likely to have developed severe pulmonary vascular disease and Eisenmenger syndrome.

Other complications
- Infective endocarditis.
- AR may develop in perimembranous and doubly committed subarterial VSDs.
- Rare risk of sinus of Valsalva dilatation and rupture with doubly committed subarterial VSDs.
- Atrial fibrillation is a late complication, associated with LA and LV dilation and dysfunction.

Physical signs
- Small restrictive VSD.
  - High-frequency pansystolic murmur loudest at L sternal edge.
- Moderate-to-large nonrestrictive VSD.
  - Displaced cardiac apex, pansystolic murmur, apical diastolic murmur, and S3 from increased flow through the MV.
- Eisenmenger VSD (see Chapter 10).

Investigation
- ECG—reflects size of shunt and presence of PAH (normal in restrictive defects).
- CXR:
  - Normal if VSD has been small from birth.
  - Moderate-sized VSD results in LV dilatation and ↑ pulmonary vascularity.
  - Eisenmenger VSD—dilated proximal PAs, oligaemic lung fields.

- Echo—identifies size, location, haemodynamic consequences, and number of defects, as well as any associated lesions.
  - Moderate-sized VSDs cause LA and LV volume overload—LA and LV dilation.
  - Large VSDs with pulmonary vascular disease cause RV pressure overload—RVH.
- Cardiac catheterization—calculate size of the shunt and pulmonary vascular resistance with reversibility studies if appropriate.

Management

Indications

- Presence of symptoms and Qp:Qs >2:1.
- Ventricular dysfunction with RV pressure or LV volume overload.
- Previous episode of endocarditis.
- Severe AR due to aortic valve prolapse into perimembranous or doubly committed subarterial VSDs.

Surgical repair

- The conducting tissue is vulnerable in perimembranous defects.
  - R bundle branch block is common after repair of pVSD.
  - Post-operative transient heart block may occur; if persists, permanent pacemaker insertion recommended due to the risk of late sudden death.
- Transatrial repair reduces risk of late RV tachycardia and dysfunction that may occur after transventricular approach.
- Long-term post-operative survival is dependent on the presence of PAH, LV dysfunction, and complications such as AR and endocarditis.

Percutaneous closure

Selected muscular and pVSDs may be device closed percutaneously in specialist centres. Particular care is required for the assessment and closure of pVSDs to avoid heart block and damage to the aortic valve.

Atrioventricular septal defects (AVSDs)

Definition
- Atrioventricular septal defects are due to abnormal development of the endocardial cushions in the embryo. They are characterized by:
  - Absent AV septum.
  - Common atrioventricular (AV) junction and AV valve ring.
  - Loss of normal 'off-setting' of the AV valves, i.e. both AV valves seen to lie at the same level on apical four-chamber view on echo.
  - The aorta is 'unwedged' from its normal position between the AV valves giving rise to a long LV outflow tract with risk of obstruction.
- The atrial component of an AVSD = ostium primum ASD.

Note
The AV valves are not true mitral and tricuspid valves and are thus termed L and R AV valves. They share five leaflets between them and are potentially regurgitant. A 'cleft' is present between the anterior and posterior bridging leaflets and is a source of regurgitation.

Types of AVSD
See Fig. 9.3.
- Partial AVSD—R and L AV valves have separate orifices; VSD is usually small or absent.
  - Cleft L AV valve.
  - >90% occur in non–Down syndrome patients.
- Complete AVSD—common AV valve and valve orifice with large VSD.
  - >75% occur in patients with Down syndrome.

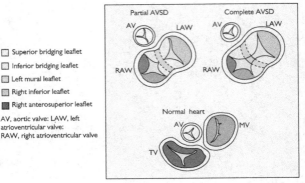

☐ Superior bridging leaflet
☐ Inferior bridging leaflet
☐ Left mural leaflet
▨ Right inferior leaflet
■ Right anterosuperior leaflet

AV, aortic valve; LAW, left
atrioventricular valve;
RAW, right atrioventricular valve

Fig. 9.3 (See also Plate 5) Schematic representation of the atrioventricular junction in AVSD. Short-axis view seen from the atrial aspect. In both forms of AVSD there is a common atrioventricular valve ring guarded by five valve leaflets. In the partial defect, the superior and inferior bridging leaflets fuse to create two separate valve orifices. This fusion does not occur in complete AVSD, so there is a common valve orifice.

Associations

- Strongly associated with trisomy 21, especially complete AVSD.
- May occur with tetralogy of Fallot and double outlet RV.

Incidence and recurrence

- $\female = \male$.
- Risk of recurrence in offspring is high—up to 10% if the mother is affected.

Clinical presentation

As for other conditions with L-to-R shunting at atrial or ventricular level, plus:

- AV valve regurgitation.
- LVOTO.
- Pulmonary vascular disease may develop if large nonrestrictive VSD.
  - Patients with Down syndrome at particular risk—coexisting upper airway obstruction, sleep apnoea, and abnormal pulmonary parenchyma may be contributory factors.

Investigation

Points to look for:

- ECG—first-degree heart block, L and superior QRS axis, notching of S waves in inferior leads.
- CXR—depends on the size of shunt and L AV valve regurgitation; cardiomegaly, LA enlargement.
- TTE—provides detailed anatomical information about the defect, degree of shunting, presence of any associated LVOTO, function and anatomy of AV valves. The absence of valvar 'off-setting' is viewed in the four-chamber view.
- Cardiac catheterization—preoperative assessment: pulmonary vascular resistance, LVOTO, acquired coronary artery disease.

Surgical management

- Partial AVSD—pericardial patch closure of primum ASD with repair of left AV valve.
- Complete AVSD—ASD and VSD repair with AV valve reconstruction. Surgical repair should not be performed if severe irreversible PAH.

Late complications post-repair of AVSD

- Recurrent AV regurgitation.
- Residual ASD or VSD.
- Residual or recurrent LVOTO.
- Complete heart block.
- Atrial arrhythmia.
- Endocarditis.

All patients require long-term follow-up due to the risk of L AV valve regurgitation, LVOTO, atrial arrhythmias, and conduction abnormalities.

Eisenmenger syndrome

Introduction

Eisenmenger syndrome can occur when there is a large, nonrestrictive communication between the systemic and pulmonary circulations. This shunt can be at atrial, ventricular, or arterial levels.

As a result of this shunt:
- High pulmonary blood flow (L-to-R shunt).
- Pulmonary vascular remodelling.
- Development of high pulmonary vascular resistance.
- Reversed or bidirectional shunt (R-to-L shunt).
- Cyanosis with PAH at systemic level.

Incidence is reducing due to improved detection of defects in infancy and availability/accessibility to surgery.

One of the most vulnerable conditions to iatrogenic complications.

Natural history

Eisenmenger syndrome is usually established in early childhood. Patients have chronic hypoxaemia and severely impaired exercise tolerance when measured objectively. They are prone to the multi-organ complications of cyanosis (see Chapter 7). Increasing age is associated with a clinical deterioration in most patients, with further reduction of exercise capacity.

Despite the chronic hypoxaemia and severe PAH, patients have a reasonable long-term prognosis: survival into the fifth decade is common, and has been reported into the eighth decade. This is in marked contrast to PAH from other causes.

Markers of poor prognosis/disease progression include:
- Complex anatomy and physiology.
- Decline in functional class.
- Heart failure.
- Arrhythmias.
- Rising serum uric acid.

Complications and extracardiac manifestations

➔ See Cyanosis, pp. 57–62.

Physical signs

- Cyanosis with clubbing.
- RV heave.
- Loud P2.
- May have pulmonary ejection click and early diastolic murmur of PR.
- No murmur from causative communication, e.g. VSD, since equal pressures on either side.
- Discriminatory signs:
  - VSD—single S2.
  - ASD—often fixed split S2.
  - PDA—normally split S2; differential cyanosis—pink fingers, blue toes.

Investigations

- ECG—p pulmonale, RVH.
- CXR—dilated proximal PAs, oligaemic lung fields.
- Echo—site of shunt, estimation of pulmonary arterial pressure, and ventricular function.
- CPEX—should be performed with caution as maximal exercise testing may induce potentially fatal syncope.
  - 6-min walk or ISWT may be better measure of exercise capacity.
- Multislice CT scanning to demonstrate:
  - Hypertensive pulmonary vasculature.
  - Collateral vessels.
  - In situ pulmonary thrombus.
  - PA aneurysms.
  - Site of any pulmonary haemorrhage.
- Cardiac catheterization is unnecessary and potentially dangerous. It should only be considered if you suspect reversibility of the high pulmonary vascular resistance which may allow surgical correction. This situation is rarely encountered in the adult population.

Management

- General measures—➔ see Cyanosis, pp. 57–62.
- Selective pulmonary vasodilators may have a role—see Chapter 16.
- Heart and lung transplantation can be considered, but is limited by complex anatomy and donor availability.

Aortic lesions

Introduction

The thoracic aortic arch is segmented into:
- Aortic root—aortic annulus to just above STJ.
- Ascending aorta—STJ to innominate artery.
- Aortic arch—innominate artery to left subclavian artery (LSCA).
- Descending aorta—LSCA to diaphragm.

Congenital anomalies can affect any segment of the thoracic aorta and are associated with significant morbidity and mortality.

Coarctation of the aorta

➲ See Fig. 11.1.

Definition and incidence
Coarctation of the aorta (CoA) is a narrowing of the aorta, usually just distal to the origin of the LSCA at the level of the duct. There is considerable variation in both the anatomy of the lesion and also the severity, which can range from mild, localized obstruction to complete interruption. Associated hypoplasia of the aortic arch is common.

Incidence
- Incidence 1:12,000 live births.
- ♂ to ♀ ratio of 3:1.
- Most commonly sporadic; rarely autosomal dominant.
- Associated with Turner's syndrome.

Associated cardiac and vascular anomalies
- Bicuspid aortic valve present in up to 80%.
- VSD.
- PDA.
- Multiple levels of left heart obstruction (see Shone syndrome, Chapter 8).
- Anomalies of head and neck vessels.
- Intracerebral berry aneurysms.

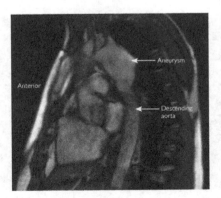

Fig. 11.1 Aneurysm post-patch repair of CoA. Sagittal section view of an MRI scan of a 25-year-old ♂ who underwent Dacron patch repair of a coarctation, age three months. He developed an aneurysm at the site of repair that expanded on serial MRI studies. He therefore underwent surgical repair of the aneurysm.

Presentation

In infancy:

Most patients with a CoA present in the neonatal period or infancy with heart failure after the duct closes. Signs include:
- Left ventricular heart failure.
- Systolic murmur.
- Reduced femoral pulses with radio femoral delay.
- Upper body hypertension.
- BP gradient between R upper and lower extremities.

In adulthood:

Less commonly, adults can present with a previously undiagnosed coarctation if either the narrowing is only mild or an adequate collateral circulation exists. The most common modes of presentation in adults are:
- Drug-resistant hypertension (most common).
- During investigation for bicuspid aortic valve disease.
- Leg claudication.
- Heart failure.
- Cerebral haemorrhage.

Physical signs

Signs to look for in adults with repaired and unrepaired CoA:
- Right-arm BP.
  - Right-arm BP will be higher than left-arm BP if the LSCA is distal to a native CoA or involved in CoA repair.
- Radiofemoral delay.
- Aortic ejection systolic murmur and ejection click from bicuspid aortic valve.
- Ejection murmur over back from CoA.
- Palpable collaterals over back in native CoA.
- Hypertensive retinopathy.

Investigations

- CXR—Fig. 11.2 shows features of unoperated CoA.
- ECG—LVH.
- Echocardiography:
  - LVH.
  - Suprasternal Doppler to assess velocity in descending aorta (peak gradient >20 mmHg with diastolic tail).
  - Associated lesions.
- MRI (➔ see Fig. 11.1).
  - Haemodynamic data.
  - 2D and 3D images of site, collaterals, and related vessels.

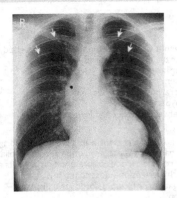

Fig. 11.2 Chest radiograph of an 18-year-old man with unoperated coarctation of the aorta and bicuspid aortic valve. There is bilateral rib notching (arrows), a dilated ascending aorta (*), and a prominent deformed aortic knuckle.

Management
- Surgical repair preferred in infants and children, with a risk of <1%. Methods include:
  - End-to-end anastomosis.
  - Subclavian flap repair (left radial pulse may be weak and left-arm BP <right-arm BP).
  - Dacron patch repair (no longer performed).
  - Bypass grafting (most common in adults).
- Transcatheter balloon dilatation and stenting is now the standard treatment for the majority of adults and older children with native CoAs or operated patients with a residual narrowing.
  - The procedure carries a risk of aortic dissection and aneurysm formation; its practice should be confined to specialist centres.

Natural history
Unoperated
The majority of adults with native CoA will die by the age of 50 years from premature coronary artery disease, stroke or aortic dissection.

Operated
The majority of patients with repaired CoA will be asymptomatic but are at lifelong risk of complications, including:
- Hypertension (incidence increases with age).
- Premature atherosclerosis.
- Complications from associated anomalies.
- Recoarctation.
- Aneurysm of repair site (most common with previous Dacron patch repair).

Follow-up

- Lifelong follow-up is required in all patients with CoA, and this should be done at a specialist ACHD clinic.
- Clinical examination, including assessment of BP and peripheral pulses, should take place every 1–2 years.
- An MRI or CT of the CoA site should be performed at a minimum of every five years; more frequently if re-CoA or aneurysm present.

Patent ductus arteriosus (PDA)

Definition
A PDA (also known as patent arterial duct) is a persistent communication between the ascending aorta and proximal LPA following birth.

Natural history and presentation in adults
Presentation depends on the size of the shunt through the PDA:
- Small—no haemodynamic significance; normal life expectancy.
- Moderate—late left heart volume overload, LV dysfunction, atrial arrhythmia.
  - Peripheral pulses may be collapsing in nature due to significant aortic run-off.
  - Continuous 'machinery' murmur.
- Large—may result in pulmonary vascular disease (Eisenmenger syndrome, see p. 113).
  - Check for differential cyanosis—blue and clubbed toes but pink fingers.

The risk of endocarditis in PDA is very small.

Management
- Closure of the PDA is recommended if clinically detectable, i.e. audible continuous murmur in L subclavian area.
- Ducts up to 14 mm in diameter are usually suitable for transcatheter closure.
- In large ducts, pulmonary vascular disease should be excluded before repair is undertaken.

Aortopulmonary (AP) window

- Rare condition.
- Direct communication between adjacent portions of proximal ascending aorta and pulmonary artery.
- Communication is usually large.
  - Physiological consequences the same as a large PDA.
- Patients surviving unoperated into adulthood are likely to have developed Eisenmenger syndrome.
- Long-term post-operative survival is good if there was low pulmonary vascular resistance at repair.

Common arterial trunk/truncus arteriosus

Definition

In this rare condition, the truncus arteriosus in the embryo fails to divide into separate aorta and pulmonary trunk. Therefore, a single great artery arises from the heart that gives rise to the coronary arteries, aorta, and pulmonary arteries. There is a single semilunar 'truncal' valve that has ≥ 3 leaflets and a subtruncal VSD.

It may coexist with interrupted aortic arch, CoA, coronary anomalies, and DiGeorge syndrome.

Management and late complications

- The majority undergo surgery within the first year of life.
  - Closure of the VSD.
  - Detachment of the PAs from the common trunk.
  - Placement of a valved RV-to-pulmonary artery conduit.
  - The truncal valve functions as the aortic valve.
- 20-year survival is >80% in patients operated in first year of life.
- Late complications are related to:
  - Truncal (aortic) regurgitation.
  - Truncal (aortic root) dilatation.
  - Ventricular dysfunction.
  - Conduit stenosis or regurgitation (multiple replacements).
  - Myocardial ischaemia (coronary abnormalities).
  - Arrhythmia.
- Unoperated, patients develop pulmonary vascular disease and Eisenmenger syndrome.

Follow-up

- Annual follow-up is recommended; it should include:
  - ECG—arrhythmia, ventricular hypertrophy.
  - Echocardiography—truncal valve function, conduit function, aortic root dimension, ventricular function, branch pulmonary artery stenosis.
- Periodically or on specific indication or suspicion:
  - Holter monitoring—suspected arrhythmia.
  - MRI—poor echocardiographic window, pre-intervention.
  - Exercise testing—functional capacity, suspected ischaemia, pre-intervention.

Marfan syndrome

Definition

Marfan syndrome is an autosomal dominant defect of connective tissue due to mutations in the gene coding for *fibrillin-1* (*FBN1*). Many mutations have been identified to date that can cause Marfan syndrome.

Diagnosis

Diagnosis is made using the revised Ghent criteria which place more weight on cardiovascular manifestations than previous criteria ——used.[1] Aortic root aneurysm and ectopia lentis are now considered cardinal features.

- Absence of family history:
  - Aortic root dilatation (Z score ≥2) or dissection and ectopia lentis.
  - Aortic root dilatation (Z score ≥2) or dissection and *FBN1* mutation.
  - Aortic root dilatation (Z score ≥2) or dissection and ≥7 points on systemic score.
  - Ectopia lentis and *FBN1* mutation.
- Family history:
  - Ectopia lentis and family history of Marfan syndrome.
  - Systemic score ≥7 and family history.
  - Aortic root dilatation (Z score ≥2 above 20 years, ≥3 under 20 years) and family history.

Management

- Patients with a dilated aorta should be commenced on a β-blocker or M angiotensin receptor blocker (ARB).
- Advise against more than mild static exercise and moderate dynamic exercise. Also avoid sports with risk of collision.
- Surgery should be considered if:
  - Aortic root dimension >50 mm.
  - Aortic root dimension >40–45 mm in high-risk situations, including females planning pregnancy or a family history of premature aortic dissection or rupture.
  - Rapid annual growth,
- A valve-sparing procedure should be encouraged.

Follow-up

Annual review is advised for all patients with Marfan syndrome and should include:

Echocardiography

- Aortic root dimensions.
- Aortic valve regurgitation.
- Left ventricular size and function.
- MV prolapse/regurgitation.

MRI

- Aortic dimensions.
- Follow-up of chronic dissection.

---

1 Loeys BL et al. 2010. The revised Ghent nosology for the Marfan syndrome. J Med Genet; 47: 476–85.

Loeys Dietz syndrome

Loeys Dietz is a connective tissue disorder first described in 2005. It shares some clinical features with Marfan syndrome but does have importance differences. It is due to mutations in the genes coding TGF-β signalling. It has autosomal dominant inheritance but there is variable expression. Up to 75 % cases are thought to be due to a new gene mutation with no family history.

Clinical features:

- Aortic aneurysms.
- Generalized arterial tortuosity.
- Hypertelorism.
- Bifid or broad uvula.
- Cleft palate.
- Cervical spine instability.
- Easy bruising and abnormal scarring.
- Uterine rupture during pregnancy and delivery.
- High risk of peripartum aortic dissection.

Diagnosis

Loeys Dietz syndrome is diagnosed through genetic testing to identify the mutation.

Management

- Annual MRI of aorta and branch vessels including head and neck.
- Baseline X-ray of cervical spine in flexion and extension.
- All patients should be on ARB regardless of the aortic size.
- Surgery should be considered if:
  - Aorta >4.5 cm.
  - Aorta >4 cm with a family history.
  - Rate of change >5 mm in 1 year.

Loeys-Dietz syndrome

Venous anomalies

Anomalies of systemic venous drainage

Introduction
Anomalies of the systemic veins are a heterogenous group of conditions and are most commonly seen as part of a complex disorder.

Superior vena cava (SVC) anomalies
Persistent LSVC
➲ See Fig. 12.1.
The commonest anomaly of systemic veins is the presence of a persistent left-sided superior vena cava (LSVC). This occurs due to failure of the LSVC to obliterate during embryogenesis.

- The LSVC drains into the right atrium via the coronary sinus in >90% of cases. A right-sided SVC is usually present too, although it may be small.
- Present in:
  - 0.3% of the general population.
  - 3% of all patients with congenital heart disease.
  - 15% of patients with tetralogy of Fallot.
- Can cause difficulty in transvenous pacing.

Diagnosis
- Echo—dilated coronary sinus (CS), opacifiction of CS on bubble contrast injection through left antecubital vein.
- CXR—LSVC may be visible.

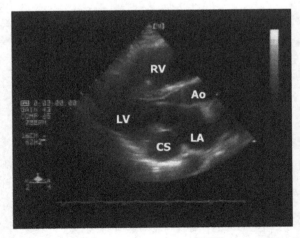

Fig. 12.1 Persistent LSVC draining to coronary sinus. 2D TTE; parasternal long axis view to show CS dilated due to receiving blood from a persistent LSVC. Ao aorta; CS coronary sinus; LA left atrium; LV left ventricle; RV right ventricle.

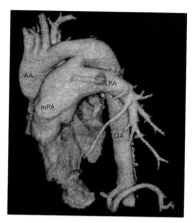

Fig. 3.20 Eisenmenger PDA. 3D reconstruction from multislice CT scan demonstrating a PDA (arrow) in a 36-year-old woman with Eisenmenger syndrome. AA ascending aorta; DA descending aorta; LPA and mPA left and main pulmonary artery.

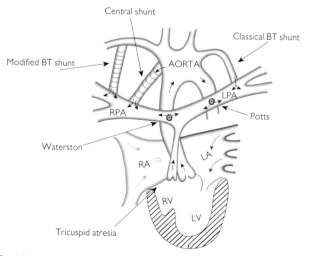

Fig. 6.2 Types of systemic-pulmonary arterial shunts (tricuspid atresia).

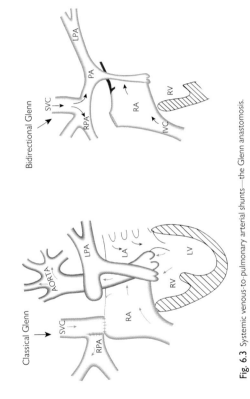

Classical Glenn

Bidirectional Glenn

Fig. 6.3 Systemic venous-to-pulmonary arterial shunts—the Glenn anastomosis.

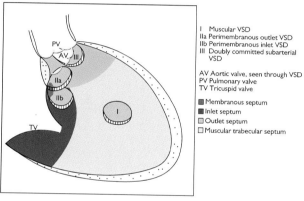

I   Muscular VSD
IIa Perimembranous outlet VSD
IIb Perimembranous inlet VSD
III Doubly committed subarterial
    VSD

AV Aortic valve, seen through VSD
PV Pulmonary valve
TV Tricuspid valve

■ Membranous septum
■ Inlet septum
☐ Outlet septum
☐ Muscular trabecular septum

Fig. 9.2 Schematic representation to show the sites of different types of VSDs. The heart is in cross-section, viewed from the R ventricular aspect.

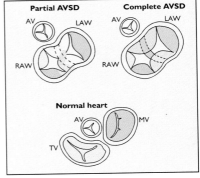

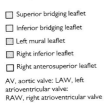

- ☐ Superior bridging leaflet
- ☐ Inferior bridging leaflet
- ☐ Left mural leaflet
- ☐ Right inferior leaflet
- ☐ Right anterosuperior leaflet

AV, aortic valve; LAW, left atrioventricular valve; RAW, right atrioventricular valve

Fig. 9.3 Schematic representation of the atrioventricular junction in AVSD. Short-axis view seen from the atrial aspect. In both forms of AVSD there is a common atrioventricular valve ring guarded by five valve leaflets. In the partial defect, the superior and inferior bridging leaflets fuse to create two separate valve orifices. This fusion does not occur in complete AVSD, so there is a common valve orifice.

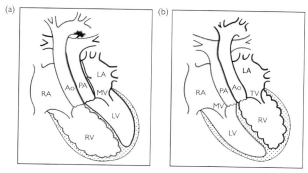

Fig. 13.1 Transposition complexes. (a) Schematic representation of complete TGA (ventriculoarterial discordance). (b) Schematic representation of ccTGA (atrioventricular and ventriculoarterial discordance). Ao aorta; LA left atrium; LV left ventricle; PA pulmonary artery; MV mitral valve; RA right atrium; RV right ventricle; TV tricuspid valve; **patent foramen ovale; *patent arterial duct.

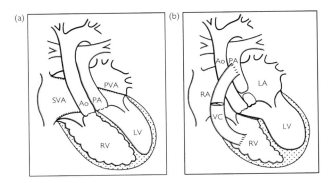

Fig. 13.2 Surgical approaches to complete TGA. (a) Schematic representation of interatrial repair (Senning or Mustard operation). (b) Schematic representation of Rastelli operation. Ao aorta; LA left atrium; LV left ventricle; PA pulmonary artery; PVA pulmonary venous atrium; RA right atrium; RV right ventricle; SVA systemic venous atrium; VC valved conduit.

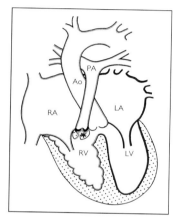

Fig. 14.1 Schematic representation of unoperated tetralogy of Fallot. *deviation of outlet septum, Ao aorta; LA left atrium; LV left ventricle; PA pulmonary artery; RA right atrium; RV right ventricle.

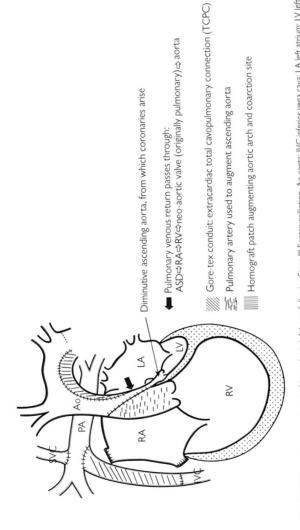

Diminutive ascending aorta, from which coronaries arise

Pulmonary venous return passes through:
ASD⇨RA⇨RV⇨neo-aortic valve (originally pulmonary)⇦ aorta

▓ Gore-tex conduit: extracardiac total cavopulmonary connection (TCPC)

▒ Pulmonary artery used to augment ascending aorta

▤ Homograft patch augmenting aortic arch and coarction site

Fig. 15.8 Schematic representation of hypoplastic left heart following Stage III Fontan palliation. Ao aorta; IVC inferior vena cava; LA left atrium; LV left ventricle; PA pulmonary artery; RA right atrium; RV right ventricle; SVC superior vena cava.

LSVC connection to LA

- Rare anomaly in which a LSVC drains directly into left atrium.
- Associated with isomerism.
- Obligatory R-to-L shunt causes cyanosis.
- Diagnosis made by L-arm bubble contrast echo.
  - Diagnosis will be missed if bubble contrast echo performed with R-arm injection.

Absent RSVC

- Rare defect that occurs in approximately 1% of patients with a persistent LSVC.
- Frequently associated with situs inversus.
- Venous blood drains to the RA via the innominate veins, LSVC, and CS.
- Unlikely to be of clinical significance except during transvenous pacing or central line insertion.

Inferior vena cava (IVC) anomaly

Azygous continuation of IVC

- Absent infrahepatic portion of IVC.
- IVC continues as azygous vein which joins the SVC in the normal position.
- Hepatic veins drain directly into the RA.
- Present in 0.6% of patients with congenital heart disease.
- Associated with complex lesions, particularly L atrial isomerism.
- Can occur in isolation and picked up as incidental finding on cross-sectional imaging or during right heart catheterization.

Diagnosis

- CXR—absence of IVC at right cardiophrenic border and dilated azygous vein.
- Cross-sectional imaging (CT or MRI).

Anomalies of pulmonary venous drainage

Total anomalous pulmonary venous drainage (TAPVD)

Definition
- Rare condition in which all four pulmonary veins drain into the right heart.
- Anomalous veins can drain directly into RA or via a common vein into a systemic vein:
  - *Supracardiac course* draining to SVC, azygous, or innominate vein.
  - *Cardiac course* draining into RA, CS, or persistent LSVC.
  - *Infradiaphragmatic course* draining to portal vein or IVC.
- Strongest predictor of poor outcome is pulmonary venous obstruction with resultant pulmonary venous hypertension and cyanosis.

Incidence and associations
- 1 in 17,000 live births.
- Obligatory R-to-L shunt to allow systemic blood flow.
- May coexist with complex cyanotic lesions and R atrial isomerism.

Natural and operated history
- 98% present in infancy with dyspnoea, cyanosis, failure to thrive.
- Symptoms due to obstruction of pulmonary venous drainage.

Operated course
- Early deaths virtually confined to those with obstructed pulmonary venous drainage.
- Excellent prognosis in surgical survivors.
- May develop obstruction of redirected pulmonary venous pathway in the growing child.
- Once fully grown, patients with no residual obstruction or associated lesions may be discharged from follow-up.

Unoperated course
- Rarely reach adulthood (only if large ASD and unobstructed pulmonary venous drainage).
- Cyanosis.
- Pulmonary vascular disease.
- Right heart failure.
- Atrial arrhythmias.

Partial anomalous pulmonary venous drainage (PAPVD)

Definition
- One or more of the pulmonary veins drain into the right heart.
- Most common variant is anomalous RUPV draining into SVC or RA (90% of cases).
- Anomalous left pulmonary veins are less common; they usually drain to left brachiocephalic or CS.

Associations
- Most commonly associated with ASDs.
  - 2% secundum ASDs.
  - 80–90% of sinus venosus ASDs.

Natural history and presentation
- Rarely symptomatic in early life if isolate lesion.
- May present in adult life, as L-to-R shunt at atrial level.
- Suspect if unexplained R heart dilatation and intact intra-atrial septum.
- Symptoms as for ASD and relate to the magnitude of the L-to-R shunt:
  - Exertional dyspnoea.
  - Atrial arrhythmias.
  - Right heart failure.
  - Pulmonary hypertension.

Diagnosis
- ECG—right bundle branch block (RBBB).
- CXR—may show abnormally draining vein.
- TTE—dilated R heart, difficult to identify PVs in adults.
- TOE—required to identify all four PVs.
- MRI—identifies anomalous PVs draining to systemic veins.

Intervention
- Indications for surgical repair same as for ASD.
- Long-term complications of repair include:
  - Obstruction of reimplanted PV—more likely if intact interatrial septum at presentation.
  - Atrial arrhythmias.
  - Obstruction of systemic venous return (very rare).

Scimitar syndrome
➔ See Fig. 12.2.
- Scimitar syndrome is a rare condition affecting 1–3/100,000 live births.
- Definition:
  - Part or all of the right-sided pulmonary veins draining to the IVC below the diaphragm via 'scimitar' vein.
  - Arterial supply of the affected right lung (usually lower lobe) from descending aorta.
  - Affected lung lobes usually hypoplastic.
- Associated cardiac lesions in 25% cases (ASD, VSD, PDA, coarctation, Fallot).

Presentation
- In adults, most commonly presents with bronchiectasis, recurrent chest infections, or haemoptysis in affected lobes.
- Exertional dyspnoea.
- Incidental CXR finding.
- Rarely causes pulmonary hypertension.
- In severe forms, associated with other lesions present in infancy, and is associated with high mortality.

Diagnosis
➔ See Fig. 12.3.
- CXR—shows anomalous pulmonary vein (said to resemble a Turkish sword or 'scimitar').
- CT or MRI—demonstrates abnormal venous drainage and arterial supply.

Management
- Intervention rarely required in adults and usually relates to the size of the shunt.
- Lobectomy or pneumonectomy may be indicated if recurrent chest infections, haemoptysis, or marked hypoplasia.

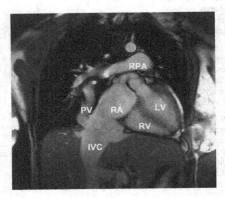

Fig. 12.2. Scimitar syndrome. Coronal section MRI scan demonstrating the anomalous RPV (that creates the 'scimitar' shape on the chest radiograph) draining to the IVC. IVC inferior vena cava; LV left ventricle; PV pulmonary vein; RA right atrium; RPA right pulmonary artery; RV right ventricle.

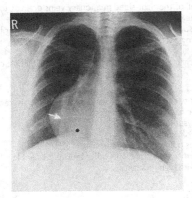

Fig. 12.3. Chest radiograph of a 25-year-old woman with scimitar syndrome. The heart is shifted into the R hemithorax because the R lung is small. The scimitar shadow (arrow) is produced by the anomalous descending venous channel which drains into the dilated IVC (*).

Transposition complexes

Introduction

Transposition complexes refer to hearts in which there is a reversal in the relationship between the ventricles and great arteries, i.e. there is ventriculoarterial discordance. Thus, the right ventricle gives rise to the aorta and supports the systemic circulation, whilst the left ventricle becomes the sub-pulmonary ventricle.

There are two types of transposition—complete transposition of the great arteries (TGA) and congenitally corrected TGA (Fig. 13.1).

Complete TGA

- Atrioventricular (AV) concordance, ventriculoarterial (VA) discordance.
  - Previously also known as D-TGA.
- Once the arterial duct and foramen ovale have closed, incompatible with life without intervention as there is complete separation of the systemic and pulmonary circulations:
  - Deoxygenated blood from the systemic veins recirculates to the aorta.
  - Oxygenated blood from the pulmonary veins recirculates to the pulmonary artery.

Congenitally corrected TGA (ccTGA)

- AV and VA discordance.
  - Previously known as L-TGA.
- ccTGA is congenitally physiologically 'corrected' since:
  - Deoxygenated systemic venous blood reaches the pulmonary artery, albeit via the morphological LV.
  - Oxygenated pulmonary venous blood reaches the aorta, but via the morphological RV.

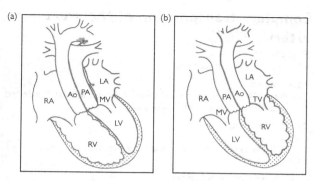

Fig. 13.1 (See also Plate 6) Transposition complexes. (a) Schematic representation of complete TGA (ventriculoarterial discordance). (b) Schematic representation of ccTGA (atrioventricular and ventriculoarterial discordance). Ao aorta; LA left atrium; LV left ventricle; PA pulmonary artery; MV mitral valve; RA right atrium; RV right ventricle; TV tricuspid valve; **patent foramen ovale; *patent arterial duct.

Complete transposition of the great arteries (TGA)

→ See Fig. 13.1(a), p. 145.
AV concordance, VA discordance.

Introduction
Complete TGA accounts for around 5% of all congenital heart disease and is more common in males than females (4:1).

Cardiac associations
- VSD in 40–50%.
- LVOTO (subpulmonary or pulmonary valvar stenosis) in up to 25%.
- CoA in 5%.

Unoperated natural history
- TGA and intact interventricular septum—only about 10% survive beyond the first year of life due to the failure of mixing of blood. Those that do survive must have mixing at the level of the atria or duct.
- TGA with VSD and PS—mixing of oxygenated and deoxygenated blood occurs at ventricular level and excessive pulmonary blood flow is prevented, resulting in a 'balanced' cyanotic circulation that may allow survival into adulthood.

Surgical management
There are three main surgical approaches to repair and the approach taken influences the long-term outcome:[1]
- Interatrial repair—Mustard or Senning operation.
- Arterial switch operation.
- Rastelli operation.

Interatrial repair—Mustard or Senning operation
→ See Fig. 13.2(a).
In an interatrial repair (or 'atrial switch') the atrial septum is excised and a saddle-shaped patch ('baffle') is placed to direct the pulmonary venous blood into the RA and RV and thence to the aorta. Systemic venous blood is directed into the LA, LV, and PA. The RV (and TV) therefore continue to support the systemic circulation.

This approach is rarely performed now and has been superseded by the arterial switch operation since the late 1980s (→ see Arterial switch operation, p. 150). However, there are many adult survivors of the approach who face inevitable late complications.

---

1 Warnes CA (2006). Transposition of the great arteries. Circulation 2006; 114(24): 2699–2709.

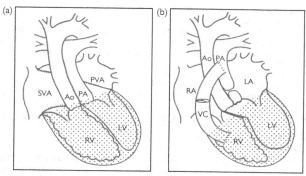

Fig. 13.2 (See also Plate 7) Surgical approaches to complete TGA. (a) Schematic representation of interatrial repair (Senning or Mustard operation). (b) Schematic representation of Rastelli operation. Ao aorta; LA left atrium; LV left ventricle; PA pulmonary artery; PVA pulmonary venous atrium; RA right atrium; RV right ventricle; SVA systemic venous atrium; VC valved conduit.

Complications of Mustard/Senning operations

- Arrhythmia—very common due to extensive atrial surgery (➔ see also Chapter 16, p. 204):
  - Bradycardia and sinus node dysfunction is often progressive.
  - Tachycardia—*atrial flutter* occurs in up to 50% of patients and incidence increases with age. It is poorly tolerated and is a likely cause of sudden death in this group of patients. Urgent DC conversion is required and subsequent referral for electrophysiology study and ablation in experienced centres should be considered.
- Sudden death is particularly common in this patient group, especially those with previous atrial flutter or poor hemodynamic status.
- Systemic (tricuspid) AV valve regurgitation.
  - Almost obligate and usually progressive.
  - TV repair or replacement should be considered before significant RV dysfunction occurs.
- Systemic (R) ventricular failure.
  - Common and progressive.
  - Associated with longstanding TV regurgitation, poor ventricular filling due to atrial surgery and myocardial perfusion abnormalities.
  - Management—standard heart failure therapy used but evidence is lacking (see Chapter 19). Optimize heart rate control as tachycardia prevents ventricular filling through the restrictive surgically modified atria.
  - Conversion to arterial switch is rarely possible beyond adolescence. See larger texts for more detail.

- Systemic or pulmonary venous pathway obstruction.
  - Few clinical signs.
  - Systemic venous pathway obstruction may be relieved by transcatheter balloon dilatation or stenting.
  - Pulmonary venous pathway obstruction usually requires surgery.
- Baffle leak
  - Occurs in up to 25% of patients.
  - Causes shunting L-to-R or R-to-L.
  - Cyanosis—increasing during exercise
  - If clinically indicated, transcatheter closure may be successful.
- PAH may develop in patients with late repair and/or associated VSD.

Arterial switch operation
➔ See Fig. 13.3.
   This is now the operation of choice in complete TGA. Blood is redirected at arterial level by switching the aorta and Pas. The coronary arteries are reimplanted into the neo-aortic root. This allows the MV and the LV to support the systemic circulation.

Complications following the arterial switch operation
- PA stenosis:
  - Common, due to stretching of the PAs to reach the neo-pulmonary trunk at the time of surgery (Le Compte manoeuvre)
  - Many require balloon dilation, stenting, or rarely reoperation.
- Coronary arteries abnormalities—rare in adulthood but obstruction of the reimplanted coronary arteries may potentially lead to myocardial infarction and sudden death.
- Neo-aortic regurgitation— usually associated with progressive neo-aortic root dilatation.

Rastelli operation
➔ See Fig. 13.2(b), p. 149.
   The Rastelli operation is performed if there is TGA plus a large subaortic VSD and PS. In this operation, the VSD is closed so that the LV empties into the aorta, the pulmonary artery is ligated, and a conduit is placed between the RV and PA. The LV therefore supports the systemic circulation.
   In the long term, there will be an inevitable need for redo conduit replacements and late risk of atrial and ventricular arrhythmias and complete heart block.

Complications following the Rastelli operation
- Conduit stenosis.
  - Inevitable need for conduit replacements. It will be possible to do some of these percutaneously.
- Atrial and ventricular tachyarrhythmias.
- Complete heart block.

Follow-up of patients with operated TGA
Most patients require annual follow-up in a specialist centre.

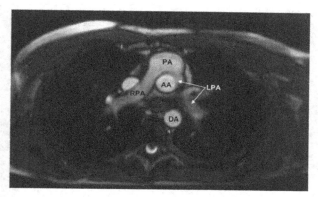

Fig. 13.3 TGA post-arterial switch operation with Le Compte manoeuvre. Transaxial MRI scan on a 19-year-old man who underwent an arterial switch operation with Le Compte manoeuvre as a neonate. The Le Compte manoeuvre involves bringing the PAs forward so that they lie anterior to, and straddle, the aorta. The LPA lies out of plane in this image. AA ascending aorta; DA descending aorta; PA, LPA, and RPA (L, R) pulmonary artery.

Examination
- Mustard/Senning:
  - Parasternal heave due to systemic RV.
  - Loud, palpable single S2 due to anteriorly lying aorta.
  - Raised JVP—PAH, baffle obstruction.
  - Congestive heart failure.
- Arterial switch:
  - Ejection systolic murmur if pulmonary artery stenosis.
  - Early diastolic murmur of AR.
- Rastelli:
  - Ejection systolic murmur of conduit stenosis.

Investigations
- ECG:
  - Senning/Mustard—may have junctional rhythm. RAD and RVH due to systemic RV.
  - Arterial switch—should be normal.
  - Rastelli—RVH indicates conduit obstruction.
- Echocardiography:
  - Mustard/Senning—patency of the systemic and pulmonary venous pathways, baffle leaks, degree of systemic AV valve regurgitation, systemic R ventricular function.
  - Arterial switch—pulmonary arterial stenoses, degree of AR, LV function. Consider stress echo if concerns about coronary perfusion.
  - Rastelli—residual VSDs, degree of conduit stenosis, LV function.

- MRI:
  - Echo rarely provides complete information in these patients; MRI is usually needed.
  - Mustard/Senning—patency of pathways, RV function, TR severity.
  - Arterial switch—pulmonary arterial stenoses, myocardial perfusion.
  - Rastelli—conduit stenosis.
- Exercise testing:
  - Useful to track objective changes in physical performance.
  - Mustard/Senning—chronotropic response to exercise (need for pacemaker), cyanosis (baffle leak or PAH).
  - Arterial switch—exercise-induced ischaemia.
- 24-hour holter monitoring—Senning/Mustard: tachy- and bradyarrhythmias.
- TOE—Mustard/Senning: useful if baffle stenosis or leaks are suspected; required during catheter intervention.

Congenitally corrected TGA (ccTGA)

→ See Chapter 12, p. 144 for description of connections and physiology and Fig. 13.1(b), p. 145.
ccTGA—AV and VA discordance

Introduction

Rare: <1% of all congenital heart disease.
- 95% have associated anomalies:
  - VSD with PS.
  - Ebstein (→ see Fig.13.4).
  - AS.
  - AVSD.
  - Abnormalities of situs.
  - Coarctation.
- 5% have congenital complete heart block that may also develop later in life.

Natural (unoperated) and operated history

Presentation will mainly depend on associated lesions. Isolated ccTGA may remain undiagnosed into old age. However, most patients develop symptoms by their fourth decade due to failure of the systemic RV, systemic AV valve regurgitation, onset of complete heart block, and atrial arrhythmias. Those with a VSD and PS may be cyanosed.

Complications of ccTGA

Systemic TV regurgitation and systemic RV failure
TR and RV dysfunction usually coexist and increase with age. RV dysfunction is associated with heart block, other cardiac lesions, and previous heart operations.
- ACE inhibitors may be useful but evidence is lacking.
- Anatomical repair (double switch or Senning-Rastelli) to restore LV to systemic circulation. This is rarely possible in adults; see larger texts for full description.
- TV replacement with a mechanical valve if RVEF ≥40%.
- Cardiac transplantation is the only option if severe TR and poor RV function and unsuitable for double-switch operation. However, pulmonary vascular resistance may be prohibitively high.

Arrhythmia
- AV block may be precipitated by surgical repair; more common with increasing age.
- Sudden death is rare in this patient group and probably related to poor ventricular function.

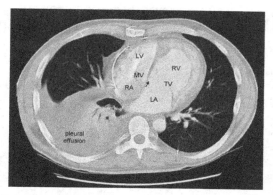

Fig. 13.4 Multislice CT scan of a 28-year-old ♂ with ccTGA. The systemic RV is dilated and hypertrophied. The interventricular septum is pushed towards the LV. There is apical displacement of the TV (arrow). The artefact across the MV is due to a pacing lead in the subpulmonary LV. There is a large R pleural effusion. LA left atrium; LV left ventricle; MV mitral valve; RA right atrium; RV right ventricle; TV tricuspid valve.

Patient assessment and follow-up

Most patients need annual follow-up in a specialist centre.

Symptoms

• Exercise intolerance, dyspnoea, palpitation, and syncope.

Clinical examination

• Parasternal heave due to the anterior systemic RV.
• Loud, palpable single S2 due to anteriorly lying aorta.
• Signs of congestive heart failure.
• TR murmur.

ECG

➔ See Fig. 13.5.

• Varying degrees of AV block or evidence of pre-excitation due to accessory pathways.
• There may be L-axis deviation.
• The R and L bundles are inverted, resulting in Q waves in V1–2 and an absent Q in V5–6 (not to be misinterpreted as a previous anterior myocardial infarction).

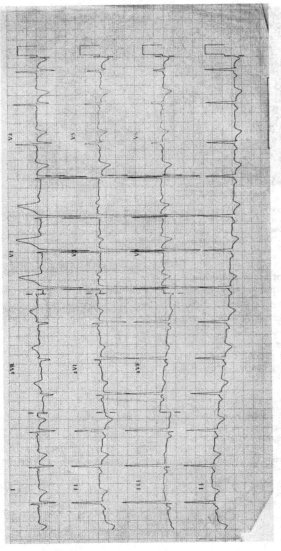

Fig. 13.5 ECG of a 30-year-old man with ccTGA. There is SR, RVH, and widespread T-wave inversion.

Echocardiography

Challenging, due to frequent cardiac malposition and discordant AV, VA connections.

- A segmental approach strongly recommended (➔ see Chapter 6).
- Assessment of systemic RV function.
- Quantitative echo-Doppler assessment of systemic (tricuspid) AV valve regurgitation is difficult; comparison with previous studies may be useful.
- Look for Ebstein-like displacement of the mural leaflet of the TV.
- Obstruction to the subpulmonary, LV outflow tract may be multi-level and PA and branches may be difficult to visualize.
- Assess associated or residual cardiac lesions.

MRI

- Complementary to echo.
- More robust method to quantify systemic RV and TV function.

Exercise testing

- Useful to track objective changes in physical performance.
- Evaluation of efficacy of medical and surgical interventions.

24-hour holter monitoring

- Progression of heart block (need for pacemaker).

Tetralogy of Fallot and pulmonary atresia with VSD

Tetralogy of Fallot

Definition
➔ See Fig. 14.1.

The primary abnormality in tetralogy of Fallot is anterocephalad deviation of the outlet ventricular septum which results in the four abnormalities described by Fallot:

- VSD.
- Subpulmonary stenosis.
- Aorta overrides crest of interventricular septum.
- Secondary RVH.

There is great morphological variation, ranging from minimal pulmonary stenosis to pulmonary atresia, and from minimal aortic override to double outlet right ventricle (DORV).

Incidence
Commonest cyanotic lesion affecting 1:3600 livebirths; ♂ = ♀.

Associations

Cardiac associations
- 16% R aortic arch (➔ see Fig. 14.2).
  - Particularly associated with 22q11 deletions.
- 15% persistent LSVC draining to CS.
  - Compared with 0.3% in general population, 3–10% in other patients with congenital heart disease.
- Secundum ASD.
- Additional VSD.
- Aortopulmonary collaterals.

Chromosome 22 deletion
- Deletion or microdeletion of chromosome 22q11.
- Associated with broad spectrum of phenotypic abnormalities, including the velocardiofacial syndrome (includes DiGeorge syndrome).
- Higher risk of recurrence of congenital heart disease in offspring if a 22q11 abnormality is present.

Abnormalities associated with chromosome 22q11 deletions
- Cardiac defects:
  - Fallot with R aortic arch.
  - Truncus arteriosus.
  - Pulmonary atresia VSD.
  - Interrupted aortic arch.
- Facial—cleft palate harelip.
- Learning difficulties and psychiatric disorder.

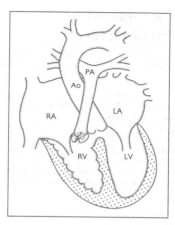

Fig. 14.1 (See also Plate 8) Schematic representation of unoperated tetralogy of Fallot. *deviation of outlet septum, Ao aorta; LA left atrium; LV left ventricle; PA pulmonary artery; RA right atrium; RV right ventricle.

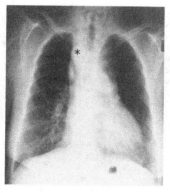

Fig. 14.2 Tetralogy of Fallot with R-sided aortic arch. Chest radiograph of a 24-year-old ♀ with repaired tetralogy of Fallot and a R-sided aortic arch (*). This anomaly is present in ~16% of patients with tetralogy of Fallot and is associated with chromosome 22q11 microdeletions.

Natural (unoperated) or shunt-palliated history

If left unoperated, only ~2% of patients survive 40 years. Survival is facilitated if there is only mild RVOTO in early life (however, this may progress over time).

Complications—unoperated

- Complications of cyanosis (➜ see Chapter 6, pp. 60–62).
- Atrial and ventricular arrhythmia.
- Progressive ascending aortic dilatation (but lower-risk dissection than that associated with Marfan syndrome).
- AR—causes volume overload of *both* ventricles and contributes to onset of biventricular failure.
- Systemic hypertension adds additional pressure overload to both ventricles and contributes to the onset of biventricular failure.
- Endocarditis.

Physical signs—unoperated

- Cyanosis, clubbing.
- RV heave.
- Palpable thrill and loud ejection systolic murmur from RVOTO.
- Soft P2.

Investigations

Points to look for:

- ECG—RAD, RVH.
- CXR— 'coeur en sabot', ↓pulmonary vascularity, may be R aortic arch.
- Echo—intracardiac anatomy and function readily identified with TTE.
- MRI—pulmonary artery anatomy, presence of collaterals.
- Cardiac catheter—PA pressure and PVR. Angiographic assessment should be made in the specialist centre prior to consideration for radical repair.

Operated history—follow-up after radical repair

 See Fig. 14.3.

Radical repair involves:
- Patch closure of VSD.
- Resection of infundibular stenosis.
- Transannular patch to enlarge pulmonary valve annulus in majority of patients.

The great majority of adults with tetralogy of Fallot have undergone radical repair. These patients have good long-term prognosis. Morbidity is likely to be better if repaired in childhood via a transatrial approach, than if repaired in adulthood or by the older transventricular approach.

All patients who have had radical repair are at risk of late complications and therefore require lifelong specialist follow-up.

Complications and sequelae of radical repair

- RBBB in >99% patients post radical repair.
  - The R bundle runs in the floor of the VSD and is damaged during surgical repair.
- Pulmonary regurgitation (PR) is an inevitable complication if repair included a transannular patch.
- Late complete heart block.
- Residual RVOTO.
- Dilated aorta.
- AR.
- Endocarditis.
- Arrhythmia (atrial and ventricular).
  - Atrial arrhythmia: ~30% under long-term follow-up. These are often scar-related intra-atrial reentry tachycardias (atrial flutter). Rapidly conducted flutter may be poorly tolerated and requires urgent cardioversion.
  - Ventricular arrhythmia: in up to 45% under long-term follow-up.
- Sudden death, likely to be arrhythmogenic.

Follow-up of the patient with severe PR

Significant PR is virtually universal if the radical repair involved a transannular patch across the RVOT. Patients are usually asymptomatic for many years, but eventually progressive RV dilation and dysfunction cause symptoms:
  - Exercise intolerance.
  - Atrial and ventricular arrhythmia.
  - RV failure.

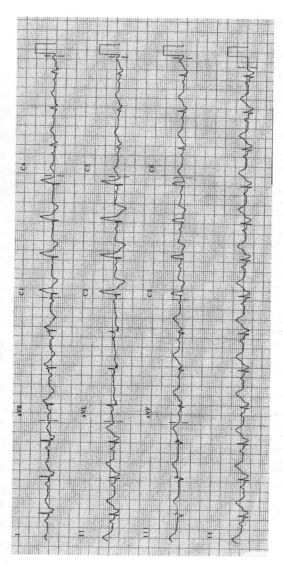

Fig. 14.3 Tetralogy of Fallot. ECG of a 22-year-old who underwent radical repair of tetralogy of Fallot aged 4. The R bundle runs in the floor of the Fallot-type VSD and is almost universally damaged at the time of surgical repair, resulting in RBBB.

Signs of severe PR
- Loss of sinus rhythm indicates decompensation—intervention is needed.
- Elevated jugular venous pressure (JVP), hepatomegaly, and peripheral oedema are all late signs indicating RV decompensation and the need for PV replacement.
- RV heave from volume-loaded RV.
- Sot P2.
- PR may be soft or inaudible (the severe regurgitant jet may be laminar and therefore inaudible).

Investigations
- ECG:
  - QRS duration: >180 ms may indicate significantly dilated RV.
  - Atrioventricular node dysfunction: heart block.
- Echo:
  - LV, RV size and function.
  - Paradoxical IVS motion.
  - Residual VSD.
  - AR.
  - Aortic root dilation.
  - RVOTO—at subvalvar, valvar, or supravalvar level.
  - Dilated CS suggesting drainage of a persistent LSVC.
- CPEX:
  - New or progressive cardiac limitation.
  - Restrictive lung defect from associated kyphoscoliosis or previous thoracotomy: may add to symptoms and increase operative risk.
- MRI:
  - Quantification of LV and RV volume and ejection fraction.
  - Quantification of pulmonary regurgitant fraction.
  - Branch pulmonary artery stenoses.
- CXR:
  - Increasing heart size.
  - Aneurysmal RVOT or PAs.
- Cardiac catheter—usually only required to relieve pulmonary arterial stenoses (balloon dilation and stent prior to surgical valve replacement).

Timing of pulmonary valve replacement
Pulmonary valve replacement should be considered if the patient has severe PR and develops:
  - Increasing symptoms, including exercise intolerance.
  - Objective impaired exercise capacity on CPEX.
  - Arrhythmias.
  - Progressive RV dilatation or dysfunction (see CMR p. 32)

Pulmonary atresia with VSD

Introduction

- Complex and heterogeneous cyanotic condition.
- Intracardiac anatomy same as in Fallot, but the RV outflow tract is blind ended (atretic).
- Pulmonary blood supply is derived entirely from three types of systemic vessels:
  - Large muscular duct that resembles a collateral.
  - Diffuse plexus of small 'bronchial' arteries arising from mediastinal and intercostal arteries.
  - Large tortuous systemic arterial collaterals—major aortopulmonary collateral arteries (MAPCAs). These arise directly from the descending aorta, its major branches, or from bronchial arteries. May connect with central PAs or supply whole segments or lobes of lung independently.

The prognosis and management depend on the pulmonary vasculature, in which there is considerable anatomical variation. Pulmonary vascular resistance depends on how many segments of lung are supplied and on the arborization pattern of the pulmonary vessels.

- If confluent PAs and MAPCAs with good arborization to all lung segments, radical repair (pink patient) possible—all MAPCAs are recruited to native PAs, place RV–PA conduit, close VSD.
- If no native PAs or unfavourable pattern of MAPCAs—no or palliative surgery possible, the patient remains cyanosed. Poor long-term outlook.

Physical signs

Similar to unoperated Fallot, plus:

- Continuous collateral murmurs.
- May have collapsing pulse.
- AR may be present.

Investigation

- CXR—R aortic arch in 25%. Typical appearance (⊃ see Fig. 14.4).
- Echo—as Fallot. Colour flow Doppler indicates collateral vessels.
- Conventional angiography in specialist centre required to precisely delineate origin, degree of ostial stenosis and intrapulmonary course of MAPCAs.
- Multislice CT and MRI useful to show relation of MAPCAs to other intrathoracic structures when planning surgery.

Late complications—unoperated or palliated

As unoperated Fallot, plus increasing cyanosis due to:

- Development of pulmonary vascular disease in lung segments perfused at systemic pressure through non-stenosed MAPCAs.
- Stenosis of MAPCAs—may be improved by stenting.

Late complications after radical repair

As repaired Fallot, plus:

- Repeated conduit replacements.
- RV failure if high pulmonary vascular resistance.

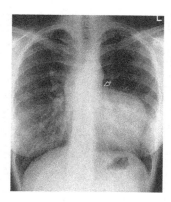

Fig. 14.4 Chest radiograph of a 21-year-old woman with tetralogy of Fallot and pulmonary atresia, no central pulmonary arteries, and multiple aortopulmonary collaterals which create an abnormal pulmonary vascular pattern. The typical 'coeur en sabot' silhouette is due to right ventricular hypertrophy and the pulmonary bay where the pulmonary artery should be (arrow). Reproduced from Warrell, D et al., (2005). Oxford Textbook of Medicine 4th edn, with permission from Oxford University Press.

Fig. 7.4 (Plate 18) A low-power photomicrograph of a section of a specimen of [text faded] and showing numerous small structures distributed throughout the tissue. The [text faded] structure is a [text faded] and surrounding this are numerous smaller [text faded] cells which form the bulk of the tissue. The specimen was prepared using standard histological techniques and stained with haematoxylin and eosin. The magnification is approximately [text faded].

Functionally univentricular hearts and Fontan circulation

The functionally univentricular heart

Introduction
Functionally univentricular hearts describes a variety of rare and complex congenital cardiac defects in which:
- There is functionally a single ventricular cavity.
- Biventricular repair is not anatomically or surgically achievable.

The ventricle may be of right or left ventricular morphology and, in the majority of cases, there is a second rudimentary nonfunctional ventricle.
   Associated abnormalities are often present including:
- Abnormal atrioventricular and ventriculoarterial connections.
- Atrial isomerism.
- Dextrocardia.
- Outflow tract abnormalities.

Common types of functionally univentricular heart
- Tricuspid atresia (rudimentary RV with dominant LV) (Fig. 15.1).
- Double inlet LV (Fig. 15.2)—often with VA discordance ± PS.
- Unbalanced atrioventricular septal defect—often associated with atrial isomerism.
- Pulmonary atresia with intact septum and hypoplastic RV (see p. 90).
- Hypoplastic left heart syndrome (Fig. 174)

Presentation
- May be diagnosed prenatally with fetal echo.
- Presentation in neonates depends on the pulmonary blood flow:
   - Too little pulmonary blood flow leads to profound hypoxaemia and circulatory collapse, requiring emergency palliation.
   - Too much pulmonary blood flow and the hypoxaemia will be less severe but child may develop congestive heart failure. If left untreated, pulmonary vascular remodelling will occur with PAH developing in early life.

Principles of management
- Physiological and anatomical considerations:
   - Correction to a biventricular circulation is not feasible.
   - All therapeutic strategies are palliative with the functionally single ventricle supporting the systemic circulation.
   - Low pulmonary vascular resistance is needed for good outcome.
   - SVC flow accounts for 70% of venous return in infant.
   - The aim of treatment is to improve cyanosis, effort tolerance, and survival.

Left untreated the natural history of univentricular hearts is very poor and few survive early childhood.

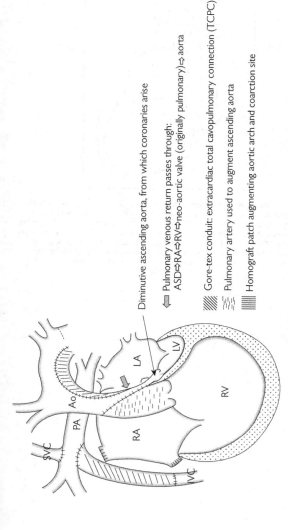

Diminutive ascending aorta, from which coronaries arise

⬇ Pulmonary venous return passes through:
ASD⇨RA⇨RV⇨neo-aortic valve (originally pulmonary)⇨ aorta

▨ Gore-tex conduit: extracardiac total cavopulmonary connection (TCPC)

▨ Pulmonary artery used to augment ascending aorta

▥ Homograft patch augmenting aortic arch and coarction site

Fig. 15.1 Schematic representation of tricuspid atresia. Systemic venous blood leaves the RA via an atrial septal defect and mixes with pulmonary venous blood in the LA. The LV thus supports both the systemic and pulmonary circulations and the patient is cyanosed. The rudimentary RV does not play a functional role. Ao aorta; LA left atrium; LV left ventricle; PA pulmonary artery; RA right atrium; RV right ventricle.

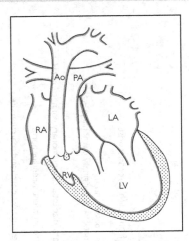

Fig. 15.2 Schematic representation of double inlet LV with VA discordance. Both atria connect to the LV via the tricuspid and mitral valves, so that systemic and pulmonary venous blood mix in the LV and the patient is cyanosed. The LV supports both the systemic and pulmonary circulations. The aorta arises from the rudimentary RV via the VSD. If the VSD is restrictive, it creates obstruction to systemic blood flow. Ao aorta; LA left atrium; LV left ventricle; PA pulmonary artery; RA right atrium; RV right ventricle; VA ventriculoarterial; VSD ventricular septal defect.

Staged approach to achieve definitive palliation

- The end result of this approach is a Fontan-type circulation (Fig. 15.3).
- Current practice is for patients to undergo a staged approach as outlined in the following sections. The number of stages will depend on the initial anatomy.
- There are many variations of the Fontan operation and this will mainly depend on timing.

Initial stage

- Initial management is to regulate the pulmonary blood flow:
  - If pulmonary blood flow is unrestricted, flow is restricted by banding the PA.
  - If pulmonary blood flow is too little (i.e. significant RVOTO), flow is augmented with a systemic-pulmonary shunt such as a modified Blalock-Taussig shunt between subclavian artery and pulmonary artery.
  - Rarely, the circulation is well balanced, and no early intervention is needed.

Cavopulmonary shunt (Glenn operation)

- Systemic venous shunt.
  - SVC is disconnected from the heart and connected directly to the PAs—a cavopulmonary anastomosis.
- This is done after 3–4 months of age when the PVR is low.
- Today, the bidirectional Glenn is used (Fig. 15.3).
  - SVC disconnected from RA; SVC connected to RPA end-to-side anastomosis; RPA left in continuity with main PA.
- Historically, a classical Glenn was performed—older patients may still have this shunt.
  - RPA disconnected from main PA; SVC disconnected from RA; SVC to RPA connected end-to-end.

Fontan operation

The final stage is the completion of the Fontan operation and is usually done around five years of age. It separates the pulmonary and systemic circulations and should abolish cyanosis. It is discussed in detail in the following sections.

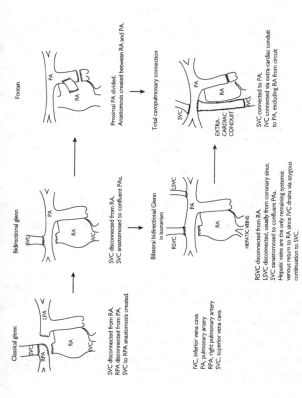

Fig. 15.3 Evolution of Fontan and total cavopulmonary connection.

Fontan circulation

General principles

- A Fontan circulation uses the functionally single ventricle to support the systemic circulation.
- The systemic venous return is directed straight into the PAs, i.e. there is no subpulmonary ventricle.
- Flow in the pulmonary circulation is therefore:
  - Passive (not pulsatile)—relies on high systemic venous pressures to provide a head of pressure to drive flow through the pulmonary vasculature.
  - Dependent on low pulmonary vascular resistance.

Types of Fontan operation

There are two main surgical approaches:

- Atriopulmonary connection—the original Fontan procedure; many variations, e.g. RA appendage connected directly to the PA.
  - Many older patients will have this type of Fontan circulation.
- Total cavopulmonary connection (TCPC):
  - Both SVC and IVC are connected separately to the PAs using a Glenn for the SVC and routing the IVC with either a lateral tunnel within the RA or with an extracardiac conduit.
  - TCPC has been the procedure of choice since ~1990.
  - The conduit is frequently fenestrated (i.e. small communication created between the Fontan circuit and the pulmonary venous atrium) to act as an escape valve for high systemic venous pressures. The result is a (small) R–L shunt that causes a degree of desaturation; however, the benefit is to offset high venous pressures and improve systemic cardiac output.

Post–Fontan surgery

See Figs 15.4–15.6.

Insert Fig. about hereThe physiological consequence of a Fontan-type operation is a circulation with high systemic venous pressures and passive pulmonary blood flow. This leads to:

- RA dilatation.
- Poor flow from atrium to PA with energy dissipation.
- Loss of effort tolerance.
- Atrial arrhythmias, often with life-threatening consequences.

Whilst the TCPC may mitigate against some of these complications, by bypassing the RA, all types of Fontan surgery rely on passive flow into PAs and produce a chronic low cardiac output state.

Physical examination

- Cyanosis and clubbing may be present if fenestration or collateral vessels.
- Pulse should be regular (check ECG).
  - Radial pulse may be absent if previous shunt.
- JVP usually is elevated ≥2 cm due to high Fontan pressures.
  - typically, CVP is ~15 mmHg compared with normal mRA pressure ~ 5 mmHg.

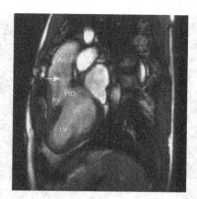

Fig. 15.4 Double inlet LV with VA discordance, post–Fontan operation. MRI scan of a 24-year-old man with double inlet LV and ventriculoarterial discordance. This sagittal section shows the anterior aorta arising from a rudimentary anterior RV. Blood passes from the LV through a large VSD. There is mild AR (arrow). The patient has undergone a Fontan procedure (not shown on this image). Ao aorta; LV left ventricle; RV right ventricle; VSD ventricular septal defect.

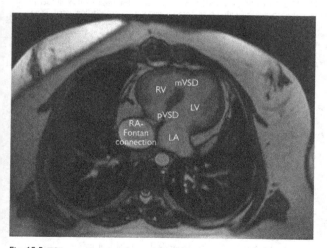

Fig. 15.5 TGA post–Fontan operation. MRI scan (transaxial view) of a 22-year-old woman with TGA, PS, straddling MV, and inlet perimembranous and muscular VSDs. The straddling MV (straddle not seen in this view) rendered biventricular repair impossible, so she underwent palliation with an atriopulmonary Fontan operation at age six. LA left atrium; LV left ventricle; mVSD muscular ventricular septal defect; pVSD perimembranous ventricular septal defect; RA right atrium; RV right ventricle.

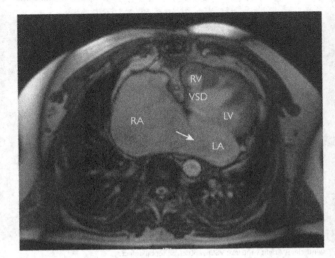

Fig. 15.6 Tricuspid atresia post–Fontan operation. Transaxial section MRI scan of a 41-year-old man with tricuspid atresia who underwent a bidirectional Glenn operation aged 10, and an atriopulmonary Fontan operation aged 21 years. There is a single atrioventricular (mitral) valve that connects to the LV. The rudimentary RV lies anteriorly. The atrial septum bows to the L (arrow) as a result of elevated pressures in the hugely dilated RA. LA left atrium; LV left ventricle; VSD ventricular septal defect; RA right atrium; RV right ventricle.

- Auscultation will not reveal murmur of underlying congenital cardiac malformation, but PSM may indicate atrioventricular valve regurgitation (AVVR).
- Often single second sound.
- May have parasternal heave if single RV.
- Normal to feel liver edge.
- Ascites or pulmonary effusion should be investigated as may be a sign of protein-losing enteropathy (PLE).
- Chest should be clear, but restrictive lung defects are common owing to previous thoracotomies.

Investigations
- ECG:
  - Check in SR.
  - May have axis deviation dependent on ventricular morphology.
  - May show atrial hypertrophy if atriopulmonary Fontan.
  - Intra-atrial reentry tachycardia may be mistaken for SR and requires prompt cardioversion (➔ see Chapter 16, p. 204).

- CXR:
  - Previous surgical procedures.
  - Kyphoscoliosis—perform lung function tests if present.
  - Indication of situs and isomerism—gas bubble, symmetry of bronchi.
- Transthoracic echocardiography:
  - Anatomy, situs and ventricular morphology.
  - Assess ventricular function.
  - Assess degree of AVVR.
  - Ventricular outflow tract obstruction.
  - Aortic incompetence.
  - Turbulent pulmonary venous return.
- Transoesophageal echocardiography:
  - Usually only performed as part of investigation of failing Fontan.
  - Evaluation of AVVR and Fontan pathway.
  - Exclude pulmonary venous obstruction.
- Cardiac MRI:
  - Assess flow in Fontan pathway.
  - Assess ventricular function and anatomy.
  - Exclude pulmonary venous obstruction.
- Metabolic exercise testing (⮕ see Chapter 3, p. 38).
  - Useful in defining the cause of exercise limitation, e.g. pulmonary or cardiac.
  - A 'good Fontan' generally has ~70% predicted MVO_2.
  - Not been evaluated in terms of prognosis in congenital heart disease.
- Blood tests:
  - FBC—Hb may be raised and platelets low reflecting cyanosis.
  - U&Es—impaired renal function is a cause for concern.
  - LFTs are often mildly deranged due to hepatic congestion. A low albumin should raise the possibility of PLE.
- Annual liver surveillance with USS and alpha fetoprotein to assess for evidence of cirrhosis and hepatic carcinoma.

Long-term complications following Fontan surgery

The risk of both cardiac and non-cardiac complications increase with age; they include:
- Atrial arrhythmias.
- SA node dysfunction.
- Systemic AV valve regurgitation.
- Ventricular dysfunction.
- Fontan pathway obstruction.
- Pulmonary venous pathway obstruction.
- Cyanosis (due to opening up of venous collaterals from the Fontan circuit to the pulmonary veins and/or flow through the fenestration).
- Development of subaortic stenosis.
- Thromboembolism.
- PLE due to high mesenteric venous pressures.
- Hepatic dysfunction and cirrhosis.
- Hepatocellular carcinoma.

Management of the post-Fontan patient

General management points

- Adult patients with an AP type Fontan should be anticoagulated with warfarin lifelong. The flow in the Fontan circuit is passive, not pulsatile, and therefore spontaneous thrombus formation is possible.
  - Protein C and S deficiency is common, further increasing the risk of thrombosis.
  - Micro thrombi in the distal pulmonary arterioles will lead to elevated pulmonary vascular resistance, detrimental to the Fontan circuit.
  - Anticoagulation in a TCPC Fontan circulation is less clear, and will vary between centres.
- Avoid dehydration:
  - Dehydration reduces the filling pressure in the Fontan circuit and reduces pre-load in the single ventricle, compromising cardiac output and systemic BP.
  - Rehydrate during intercurrent illness.
  - If nil by mouth (NBM), give IV fluids, 1 L normal saline over 12 hours.
- GA:
  - Senior advice should be sought early on.
  - Hydrate with IV fluids when NBM.
  - All anaesthetic agents cause systemic vasodilatation.
  - Positive pressure ventilation further reduces venous return and therefore cardiac output.
  - Lack of pre-load recruitment makes low systemic vascular resistance (SVR) difficult to overcome.
  - Have metaraminol available to maintain SVR and systemic BP during anaesthesia.
- Atrial flutter/tachycardia (➲ see also Chapter 16, p. 204, and Fig. 15.7):
  - A common and life-threatening event, especially with advancing age.
  - Mechanism is a scar-related intra-atrial reentrant tachycardia (IART) or atypical atrial flutter.
  - Rhythm is usually regular and often not rapid (HR 90–120).
  - ECG may be mistaken for SR—compare with ECG in normal sinus rhythm (ensure patients carry a copy of their normal ECG at all times).
  - Do not attempt chemical cardioversion as may trigger rapid conduction and circulatory collapse.
  - Arrange prompt cardioversion.
  - All Fontan patients who have had an episode of atrial flutter should be discussed with an electrophysiologist with expertise in this patient group. An EP study and ablation may be appropriate to reduce the risk of further episodes—check that there is access to the heart.
  - Long-term prevention with amiodarone may be necessary (check thyroid function every three months: thyrotoxicosis is a common late side effect, which may cause permanent deterioration in functional status).

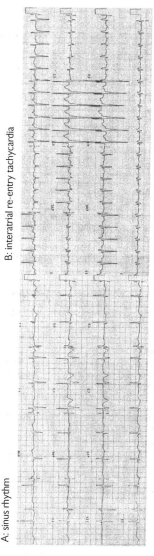

A: sinus rhythm

B: interatrial re-entry tachycardia

Fig. 15.7 Atrial tachyarrhythmia post-Fontan operation for tricuspid atresia.

A 24-year-old man who underwent Fontan palliation for tricuspid atresia in childhood had episodes of interatrial tachyarrhythmia. 12-lead ECG (a) shows him in sinus rhythm. He had been advised to seek urgent medical assistance if he developed palpitation. He began to feel unwell and breathless with palpitation, but delayed for two days before presenting to a local emergency department. His ECG (b) showed an IART but was misdiagnosed as sinus tachycardia and no treatment was given. The following day he had a cardiac arrest and could not be resuscitated. At-risk patients should be advised to seek help rapidly if palpitation occurs, and given copies of their ECGs to carry, along with a letter detailing their diagnosis and instructions for emergency cardioversion.

The failing Fontan

Definition
- Without Fontan-type surgery, the majority of single-ventricle patients would not survive into adulthood.
- A Fontan circuit is by its nature palliative.
- The Fontan circulation is a chronically low cardiac output state.
- Effort tolerance is limited even in 'well' patients.
- Signs of 'failure' include:
  - Ventricular dysfunction.
  - Reduced effort tolerance.
  - Arrhythmias.
  - PLE.

Why it happens
Ventricular dysfunction
- Increased afterload leads to hypertrophy of ventricle.
- Limited pre-load recruitment leads to diastolic dysfunction.
- Ventricular hypertrophy leads to systolic dysfunction.
- Management:
  - No data to support conventional therapy, e.g. ACE inhibitors, beta-blockade, spironolactone.
  - Evidence emerging from small studies that selective pulmonary vasodilator drugs, such as sildenafil and bosentan, may improve ventricular dysfunction and functional class (see Chapter 19, Heart failure).
  - O_2 therapy may help.
  - Diuretics should be used with caution due to risk of hypovolaemia.
  - Exclude underlying causes, e.g. outflow tract obstruction, AVVR, Fontan pathway obstruction, pulmonary venous obstruction, paroxysmal arrhythmias.

Reduced effort tolerance
- Impaired ventricular function.
- AVVR, often due to annular dilatation; leads to increased atrial pressure.
- This further reduces the effective gradient down which blood flows and thus further reduces the cardiac output.
- Management:
  - Ensure no respiratory contributing factors.
  - A prescribed exercise program may improve symptoms of breathlessness and improve exercise capacity.

Pulmonary vascular remodelling
- Distal muscularization of pulmonary arterioles occurs leading to:
  - ↑ pulmonary vascular resistance.
  - ↓ flow through lungs.
  - Failure to pre-load recruit, which in turn leads to lower cardiac output.

- Management:
  - Impossible to prove without lung biopsy (*not* recommended).
  - Empiric therapy with targeted pulmonary vasodilator therapy may help, but to date, evidence is available only for small, single-centre studies and case reports.

Atrial arrhythmias
- Multiple scars, related to suture lines and bypass cannulation, provide circuits for macro-reentrant tachycardias.
- Increasing incidence with age.
- Associated with decline in ventricular function.
- Management:
  - See previous discussion.

PLE
- Particular problem for Fontan patients.
- High mesenteric venous pressure leads to protein loss into the gut.
- Assessed by demonstrating low serum albumin and immunoglobulins and raised faecal alpha-1 antitrypsin levels from a fresh stool sample (contact local biochemistry department for details of sampling).
- Low albumin, total protein and immunoglobulin levels leads to effusions, ascites, dependent oedema, malnutrition, recurrent cellulitis, and septicaemia.
- No reliably effective treatment; *may* benefit from:
  - Daily unfractionated SC heparin.
  - Oral budesonide.
  - Targeted pulmonary vasodilator therapy.
  - Fenestration of Fontan pathway.
- 50% five-year mortality—seek expert help early if suspected.

Long-term outcome of Fontan surgery
- The long-term outcome is not known.
- Current adult patients are the pioneers of this operation.
- Complications, as already discussed, will inevitably cause significant morbidity and mortality.
- Fontan patients form a small proportion of the total number of patients with congenital heart disease, but account for 50% of emergency admissions.
- Prompt management of their medical emergencies will reduce the risk of premature death.

Hypoplastic left heart syndrome

Hypoplastic left heart syndrome (HLHS) includes a range of cardiac conditions in which there is stenosis, hypoplasia, or atresia at different levels of the left heart. HLHS includes severe aortic stenosis/atresia, mitral atresia, and unbalanced AVSD. This results in a small left ventricle that is unable to support the systemic circulation and a diminutive aorta which gives rise to the coronary arteries.

HLHS accounts for 2% of all congenital cardiac lesions.

Presentation

- Detected *in utero* or shortly after birth when the duct closes, leading to cardiovascular collapse.
- Not compatible with survival unless operated.

Surgical management

In infancy, patients undergo multistage repair, termed a Norwood repair, first described in 1983.

Stage I

- Performed in first few days of life.
- The systemic outflow tract and aorta are reconstructed using the right ventricle and main pulmonary artery (Damus-Kaye-Stansel procedure).
- Pulmonary blood flow is provided through a systemic-pulmonary shunt (Blalock-Taussig) or, in recent modifications of the operation, an RV–PA conduit.
  - Placement of RV–PA conduit improves systemic and coronary perfusion because there is no diastolic coronary run-off; as well, growth of the branch PAs improves due to pulsatile flow.

Stage II

- Performed at 4–6 months.
- Cavopulmonary/Glenn shunt and take down of systemic shunt/conduit.

Stage III

See Fig. 15.8.
- Performed between 3–5 years.
- Completion of a Fontan circulation, usually an extracardiac conduit.

Natural history

- Around 70% of patients undergoing Norwood repair now reach adulthood.
- Long-term complications are those of any Fontan, plus:
  - Coarctation repair site—recoarctation?
  - LPA—stenosis?
  - ASD—restrictive?
  - Coronaries from diminutive aorta—ischaemia?
  - Systemic RV—dysfunction?
  - Systemic tricuspid valve—regurgitation?

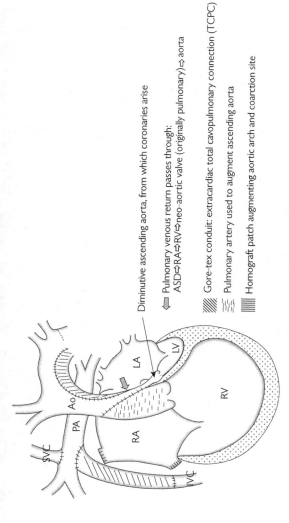

Diminutive ascending aorta, from which coronaries arise

Pulmonary venous return passes through:
ASD⇒RA⇒RV⇒neo-aortic valve (originally pulmonary)⇒aorta

Gore-tex conduit: extracardiac total cavopulmonary connection (TCPC)

Pulmonary artery used to augment ascending aorta

Homograft patch augmenting aortic arch and coarction site

Fig. 15.8 (See also Plate 9) Schematic representation of hypoplastic left heart following Stage III Fontan palliation. Ao aorta; IVC inferior vena cava; LA left atrium; LV left ventricle; PA pulmonary artery; RA right atrium; RV right ventricle; SVC superior vena cava.

Pulmonary hypertension in ACHD

Introduction

Pulmonary arterial hypertension (PAH) is a common complication in patients with ACHD, with a prevalence of around 10% in developed countries. It is most commonly due to large, uncorrected left-to-right shunts, although a permissive genotype might explain its development in other, seemingly lower-risk, patients. Histologically, PAH in ACHD is the same as PAH due to other aetiologies, such as idiopathic and connective tissue disease. There is progressive endothelial dysfunction, vasoconstriction, and pulmonary vascular remodelling due to an imbalance of vasoactive substances, including prostacyclin, nitric oxide, and endothelin-1.

The development of PAH in this patient group has a significant impact on both morbidity and mortality, and should be managed in specialist centres with both ACHD and PAH expertise.

Classification

As shown in Table 16.1, the European Society of Cardiology (ESC) has classified patients with PAH secondary to ACHD into four groups depending on their underlying anatomy and physiology.[1]

Table 16.1 ESC classification of patients with PAH

Group A	Eisenmenger syndrome
Group B	PAH associated with systemic-pulmonary shunts*
Group C	PAH associated with small defects**
Group D	PAH following corrective surgery

*Moderate and large shunts, still predominantly left-to-right, no cyanosis at rest

**VSD <1 cm, ASD <2 cm—behave like idiopathic PAH, defects may be coincidental

1 Galie N, Hoeper M, Humbert M, et al. Guidelines for the diagnosis and treatment of pulmonary hypertension. Eur Heart J 2009; 30(20): 2493–2537.

Investigations

- ECG:
  - Evidence of right heart strain.
- CXR:
  - Prominent main pulmonary arteries, cardiomegaly.
- Echocardiogram:
  - Estimation of PASP from maximal tricuspid regurgitation velocity (Table 16.2).
  - Dilated right-sided chambers.
  - Impaired right ventricular function.
  - Right ventricular hypertrophy.
  - Abnormal interventricular septal motion.
  - RVOT acceleration time <120 ms corresponds to elevated PA pressure.
- 6-minute walk/incremental shuttle walk test.
- Right heart catheter:
  - Perform if non-invasive screening suggests a diagnosis of PAH and ASD or left-to-right shunt.
  - Not usually required for diagnosis in established Eisenmenger syndrome because the diagnosis can be made non-invasively and catheterization is associated with significant risk.
  - Direct measurement of mean PA pressure, RA pressure, PCWP.
  - Allows calculation of cardiac output (CO) and pulmonary vascular resistance (PVR):

$$PVR = \frac{MPA - PCWP}{CO}$$

Table 16.2 Likelihood of PAH from echocardiographic estimations of PASP

Estimated PASP on echo (mmHg)	Likelihood of established PAH
≤36	Unlikely
≤36 + other features of PAH	Possible
37–50	Possible
>50	Likely

Management

General

- Encourage active lifestyle whilst keeping within own abilities and avoiding strenuous activities.
- Annual flu vaccination.
- Avoid routine venesection and maintain optimum iron stores.
- Effective contraception (avoid oestrogen-containing preparations).
- Oxygen can be used for symptomatic benefit but has not been shown to affect survival.

Advanced targeted therapies

Advanced therapies include endothelin antagonists such as bosentan, ambrisentan, macitentan, and phosphodiesterase-5 (PDE-5) inhibitors, such as sildenafil and tadalafil. They are widely used in patients with Eisenmenger syndrome in functional class III or IV. The BREATHE-5 trial showed a reduction in PVR and an increase in 6-minute walk distance and functional class after 16 weeks of bosentan therapy. Similar results have been shown with PDE-5 inhibitors.

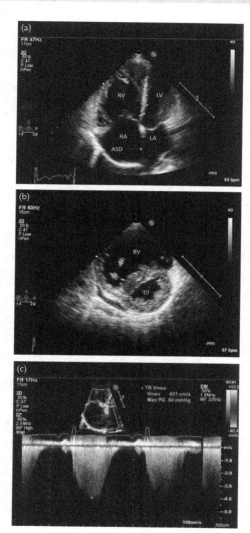

Fig. 16.1 TTE of 34-year-old man with severe pulmonary hypertension secondary to a large ASD showing (a) dilated and hypertrophied RV with ASD, (b) RVH with flattening of interventricular septum, (c) Estimated TR V_{max} 64 + RAPmmHg suggesting established PAH highly likely.

Rare conditions presenting in adulthood

Coronary anomalies

Coronary anomalies are rare but important to consider as they have the potential to impair myocardial blood flow, leading to ischaemia, arrhythmias, and sudden death. They can occur in isolation or in association with other congenital cardiac lesions.

The main types of coronary artery anomalies are outlined in Table 17.1. Ischaemia is the main indication for surgical repair; it is associated with:

- Anomalous proximal coronary course between aorta and pulmonary trunk.
- An intramural proximal segment of the anomalous coronary artery inside the aortic wall.
- Acute angulation between origin of anomalous coronary artery and the aortic wall.
- Anomalous coronary artery arising from pulmonary trunk.

Left coronary artery from pulmonary artery (LCAPA)

- Rare anomaly that most commonly presents in infancy with myocardial ischaemia and LV failure when pulmonary vascular resistance decreases.
- 10–15% survive into adulthood due to the development of an adequate intercoronary collateral circulation.
- Adult presentation:
  - Asymptomatic.
  - Myocardial ischaemia or MR due to papillary muscle dysfunction.
- Surgical repair indicated.
- Post-surgical survival related to the amount of ischaemic damage and the degree of MR.

Congenital coronary arteriovenous fistulae

- The coronary arteries have a normal origin, but there is a fistulous coronary artery branch communicating directly with RV in 40%, RA in 25%, PA 15%, rarely SVC or PV.
- Survival into adulthood is usual.
- Longevity reduced if the communication is large and leads to coronary steal phenomenon and myocardial ischaemia.
- Increased incidence of symptoms with age:
  - Endocarditis.
  - Heart failure.
  - Arrhythmia.
  - Myocardial ischaemia and infarction.
  - Sudden death.
- Surgical repair recommended unless trivial isolated shunt.
- Some smaller fistulae may be amenable to transcatheter device occlusion.

Table 17.1 Major types of coronary anomaly

Anomalous origin from inappropriate aortic sinus or coronary vessel	LMS: absent (separate origins of LAD and Cx)
	LAD: from R aortic sinus or RCA
	Cx: absent, or from R aortic sinus or RCA
	RCA: from L or posterior aortic sinus, or LAD
	Single coronary artery from R or L aortic sinus
Anomalous origin from other systemic artery (rare)	Innominate, subclavian, internal mammary, carotid, bronchial arteries, or DA
Anomalous origin from PA	
Coronary arteriovenous fistulae	

Cx circumflex; DA descending aorta; LAD left anterior descending; LMS left main stem; PA pulmonary artery; RCA right coronary artery.

Investigations

Congenital anomalies should be considered in adults <50 years with symptoms of ischaemia, impaired LV, or MR secondary to papillary muscle dysfunction. Investigations should include the assessment of:

- Ischaemia—functional imaging to induce ischaemia, 24-hour ECG tape to assess for arrhythmias.
- Anatomy—selective angiography and multislice CT may be required to delineate precise course of anomalous vessels.

Sinus of Valsalva aneurysm

Definition and natural history

- Dilatation or enlargement of ≥1 of the aortic sinuses.
- Unruptured aneurysm rarely symptomatic, but may cause obstruction—chest pain, palpitation.
- Aneurysm may progress and rupture:
  - Non-coronary sinus usually into RA.
  - R coronary sinus into RA or RV.
- Rupture usually in early adulthood, sometimes precipitated by endocarditis:
  - Tearing chest pain, dyspnoea, heart and renal failure, loud *continuous* murmur.
  - Small perforations may be asymptomatic.

Management

Unruptured

- Monitor with yearly echo if asymptomatic.
- If causing symptoms, surgical repair.

Ruptured

- Diagnosis clinical—typical history and murmur.
- Confirm site with echo and angiography.
- Surgical or transcatheter repair required.

Part 3

General management issues of adult congenital heart disease

Emergencies

Introduction

There are a number of ACHD emergencies in which quick and simple management can prevent unnecessary morbidity or mortality. Senior in-house
help must always be requested and urgent advice sought from the specialist
ACHD unit.

Haemoptysis in a cyanotic patient

→ See also Chapter 6, pp. 58–62.

Haemoptysis is one of the leading causes of death in cyanotic patients,
especially in the presence of pulmonary hypertension. The specialist ACHD
centre should be liaised with early as urgent transfer may be required.
Always establish the patient's diagnosis and any recent intervention or
surgery.

The principles of management are:
- Resuscitate the patient with an ABC approach.
- Gain IV access and give maintenance IV fluids through an air filter to
  prevent paradoxical embolism through a R-to-L shunt.
- Send bloods for FBC, clotting, X-match.
  - Remember that the INR may be spuriously raised if high haematocrit
    (use a citrate-depleted bottle if available).
- Keep patient NBM.
- Lower the systemic BP if necessary:
  - Remember that brachial artery pressure = PA pressure in
    Eisenmenger syndrome.
  - Important to lower pressure in bleeding pulmonary vessel.
  - IV beta blockers if appropriate.
  - Avoid vasodilating agents that will increase the R-to-L shunt and thus
    exacerbate the hypoxia.
- If severe haemoptysis, consider selective intubation.
- Give opiates and/or benzodiazepines if significant bleed to reduce
  patient's distress; this will also lower blood pressure.
- Consider an urgent CT scan—involve the congenital interventional
  cardiologist; there may be a vessel to embolize or coil.

Possible causes of haemoptysis

This will depend on anatomy, but can include:
- Embolism of *in situ* PA thrombus; pulmonary embolism from other
  sources such as DVT is unlikely.
- Bleeding from pulmonary arteriovenous malformations.
- Bleeding collateral vessels.
- Chest infection.

Other emergencies and pitfalls to avoid in cyanotic heart disease

➔ See Chapter 6, pp. 56–62.
- Avoid:
  - Dehydration—give IV fluids through a filter if patient NBM.
  - Iatrogenic renal failure—e.g. contrast agents, aminoglycosides, NSAIDs.
  - Paradoxical embolism.
  - Increasing cyanosis with vasodilators.
- Maintain appropriately high haemoglobin for optimum O_2-carrying capacity—a 'normal' haemoglobin in a cyanotic patient suggests significant iron deficiency and will compromise the patient's O_2-carrying capacity.
- Rapid recognition and management of tachyarrhythmias (see following).
- Management of cerebral abscess.

Haemoptysis or haematemesis in patients with repaired coarctation

➔ See also Chapter 10, pp. 118–21.
- Assume that any haemoptysis or haematemesis in these patients represents an aorto-bronchial or aorto-oesophageal fistula due to the erosion of an aortic aneurysm.
- Highest risk in patients who have had a Dacron patch repair of their coarctation, as aneurysms develop at the suture lines.

Management
- Resuscitate the patient with a ABC approach.
- IV access.
- Send bloods for FBC, clotting, and X-match.
- Keep patient NBM.
- Arrange an urgent contrast CT or MRI scan.
- Avoid invasive tests (bronchoscopy, upper GI endoscopy, aortography) due to risk of causing catastrophic haemorrhage.
- Liaise with specialist ACHD centre—patient needs urgent transfer for emergency surgery or aortic stenting.

Tachyarrhythmias

⤷ See Fig. 18.1.
- Patients with congenital heart disease are at increased risk of tachyarrhythmias due to:
  - Surgical scars (both atrial and ventricular).
  - Chronic pressure or volume overload.
  - Chronic hypoxia.
  - Defects giving rise to ischaemia.
  - Associated anomalies, e.g. accessory pathways in Ebstein anomaly.
- Tachyarrhythmias can be poorly tolerated by certain patient groups, particularly those with a Fontan circulation or previous atrial switch (see following), or those with impaired ventricular function. These patients therefore need *urgent* DC cardioversion, *not* pharmacological therapy which is potentially lethal.
- Common precipitating factors for atrial arrhythmias include:
  - Alcohol.
  - Drug abuse.
  - Fatigue.
  - Unaccustomed overexertion.
  - Thyrotoxicosis (beware amiodarone).

Why atrial tachyarrhythmias are so dangerous

TGA with atrial switch (Mustard/Senning) (⤷ Chapter 12, p. 148)
- Flutter increasingly common with age and ventricular dysfunction.
- Restrictive atrial pathways mean that ventricular filling is compromised at rapid heart rates.
- Flutter may conduct 1:1—a heart rate of 300 bpm may be fatal in this group.
- Failure to give IV fluids or giving IV antiarrhythmics may cause cardiovascular collapse from which patient cannot be resuscitated.

Fontan (⤷ Chapter 14, p. 171)
- IART (atypical flutter) is common, especially in atriopulmonary Fontan with dilated RA.
- The Fontan circulation relies on a very small pressure gradient across the pulmonary circulation, permitting systemic venous blood to cross the pulmonary vascular bed into the LA and then into the ventricle. During flutter, the LA pressure rises and impedes blood flow into the ventricle → cardiac output falls.
- If mismanaged, flutter may be fatal:
  - If no IV fluids are given, the systemic venous pressure falls, further reducing forward flow across the pulmonary circulation → cardiac output falls further.
  - Antiarrhythmics, e.g. IV beta blockers and flecainide, are unlikely to cardiovert the patient, but may produce profound hypotension → cardiac output falls.

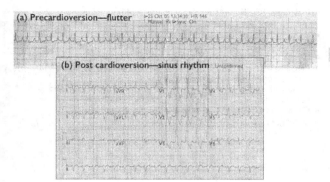

Fig. 18.1 Atrial flutter post–Mustard repair of TGA. A 26-year-old ♂ who underwent Mustard repair of TGA in infancy presented hypotensive to the emergency department with syncopal palpitation of three hours' duration. The rhythm strip (a) shows atrial flutter with 2:1 block. He reverted to sinus rhythm with urgent DC cardioversion; (b) there is R axis deviation and R ventricular dominance.

DC cardioversion in Fontan patients
- When cardioverting these patients, vasodilator anaesthetic agents should be given cautiously due to slow circulation time.
  - Vasodilatation will further reduce systemic venous pressure → cardiac output falls.
- Positive pressure ventilation raises intrathoracic pressure and reduces systemic venous return still further → cardiac output falls → and patient cannot be resuscitated.

Patient-carried ECGs
Patients with complex congenital heart disease often have very abnormal baseline ECGs, and interpreting them in an emergency can be difficult. Failure to recognize loss of sinus rhythm can result in the patient dying.

All patients with congenital heart disease and abnormal resting ECGs should be given a copy of their baseline ECG to carry on their person, so that the admitting team can compare it with the admission ECG.

Management of atrial flutter/ventricular tachycardia
- Resuscitate the patient with an ABC approach.
- If patient is compromised, urgent DC cardioversion (ALS protocol).
- IV access and start IV fluids through an air filter.
- Send bloods for K⁺, Mg²⁺, TFTs, C-reactive protein (CRP), FBC, biochemistry, and INR.
- Move to CCU and monitor whilst arranging DC cardioversion.
- Inform senior cardiology and specialist ACHD centre.

- May need TOE if INR subtherapeutic or >24 hours' duration (AF/flutter), but do not delay cardioversion if patient compromised.
- Liaise with senior anaesthetist (preferably cardiac)—need to inform about cardiac anatomy and physiology and need for urgency.
- DC cardioversion (external pads) as ALS protocol.
- Need to monitor following cardioversion for at least six hours and investigate the reason for arrhythmia.
- Liaise with specialist ACHD centre re: discharge medication and consideration of ablation referral/further investigation.
- Obtain old ECGs and give patient copy of arrhythmia and discharge ECG.

Heart failure in ACHD

Introduction

Despite the advances in surgical techniques, only very few patients with CHD are have a truly curative procedure, with the majority of patients being at lifelong risk of complications including ventricular dysfunction, arrhythmias, and premature death. Ventricular dysfunction, leading to heart failure, remains a major cause of both morbidity and mortality, with some studies showing that it accounts for up to 40% of deaths in adults with CHD.

Factors associated with ventricular dysfunction include:
- Longstanding volume overload.
- Longstanding pressure overload.
- Cyanosis.
- Surgical insult.
- Systemic right ventricle.
- Single-ventricle physiology (especially if morphologically right ventricle).

Drug therapy

Patients with ACHD were excluded from most chronic heart failure drug trials. Physicians frequently apply knowledge gained from acquired heart failure to these patients. ACHD patients, however, have unique anatomical and physiological abnormalities, and should be considered a different population.

- Drug trials in ACHD:
  - Small patient numbers.
  - Frequently single-centre.
  - Often use surrogate end points.

Two groups who highlight specific difficulties are those with a systemic right ventricle (atrial switch, ccTGA) and those with a univentricular heart, including those with a Fontan circulation. The use of standard heart failure treatment remains unclear in these patient groups and needs large, multi-centre trials.

- ACE inhibitors/ARBs:
  - Lack of evidence to date for any improvement in ventricular function, quality of life, or exercise capacity in patients with systemic RVs or univentricular hearts.
- Beta blockers:
  - Improvement in functional class demonstrated in systemic RVs along with an increase in ejection fraction in univentricular hearts.
- Aldosterone antagonists:
  - A reduction in myocardial fibrosis has been demonstrated, but this has not been associated with any functional improvement.
- Selective pulmonary vasodilators:
  - In patients with a Fontan circulation, several small, single-centre studies have demonstrated improvement in functional class and measures of ventricular function with both the endothelin antagonist, bosentan, and PDE-5 inhibitor, sildenafil.

Transplantation in ACHD

As survivors with complex ACHD increase, there will be an inevitable increase in patients with end-stage heart failure who have no further conventional medical or surgical options. For these patients, heart or heart-lung transplantation may be the only remaining treatment to improve survival and quality of life. Despite increasing numbers of transplants performed in patients with ACHD, numbers remain relatively small. Patients should therefore ideally be managed in large centres with the appropriate expertise and experience.

• Specific problems associated with this patient group when considering transplantation include:
  • Complex anatomy.
  • Multiple previous operations.
  • ↑ PVR.
  • HLA sensitization (especially if previous homograft).
  • Very heterogeneous population.
  • Criteria for referral not always well defined → patient listed too late.
• As a result of these problems:
  • Patients wait longer on waiting list for an organ.
  • Longer intraoperative ischaemic time.
  • Worse 30-day survival compared to acquired heart failure but comparable long-term survival.

End-of-life care in ACHD

With increased survival of adults with congenital heart disease, there will be an increasing number of patients with advanced disease who will require end-of-life (EOL) care. A proactive approach around EOL discussions has been shown to be beneficial to patients with cancer and acquired heart failure. Whilst heart failure is the most common cause of death in ACHD, sudden cardiac death still accounts for a significant number and thus it is not appropriate to wait for heart failure to develop before starting these conversations.

Specific difficulties around this in patients with ACHD include:
• Population of patients previously heralded as a success story of cardiac surgery → change from a life-prolonging to palliative approach.
• Outlook and survival often unclear and unpredictable.
• Lifelong illness and frequently no trigger for deterioration making it difficult to judge when to discuss.
• Often young patients with unique needs may act as a further barrier to communication.
• Difficult balance between life-prolonging interventions, including transplantation, and EOL care.

Discussion and planning of EOL issues should become a routine part of our patients' assessment, and a proactive approach is needed for this to happen. Furthermore, this should be re-evaluated at every significant clinical change.

Device therapy in ACHD

Introduction

Conduction disease and arrhythmias cause substantial morbidity in adults with congenital heart disease. The clinical significance can vary from benign to potentially life-threatening. The substrates for these include underlying developmental abnormality (ccTGA, left atrial isomerism, Ebstein anomaly), scar tissue within atria/ventricles due to previous surgery (tetralogy of Fallot, Fontan, atrial switch for TGA), and consequences of significant haemodynamic lesions (e.g. severe PR following repaired Fallot).

Insertion of devices in these patients requires special consideration. Knowledge of underlying anatomy, previous surgical procedures, and vascular access routes is crucial; equally important is an understanding of problems likely to be encountered with lead placement in complex hearts and obtaining a stable position. Most problems can be avoided by careful pre-procedural planning, especially in the more complex hearts, e.g. Fontan and atrial switch.

Bradycardia pacing

Indications[1]

Class I

- Symptomatic sinus node disease, including sinus bradycardia and chronotropic incompetence.
- Congenital AV block + wide QRS escape rhythm, complex VEs, or ventricular dysfunction.
- Second- or third-degree AV block.
- Ventricular arrhythmias due to AV block.

Class IIa

- Impaired haemodynamics due to sinus bradycardia or AV block.
- Sinus or junctional bradycardia to reduce risk of IART.
- Congenital AV block resting daytime HR <50 bpm.
- Complex CHD + sinus/junctional bradycardia with awake HR <40 bpm or pauses >3 s.

Class IIb

- Moderate CHD + sinus/junctional bradycardia with awake HR <40 bpm or pauses >3 s.
- Transient post-op AV block + bifasicular block.

Special anatomical considerations for pacing in ACHD

Simple lesions—ASDs/VSDs

- If repaired, generally straightforward lead placement—surgical patches may make optimal lead placement difficult.
- If unrepaired, consider pre-device defect closure, alternative lead placement (e.g. epicardial), or concomitant anticoagulation.

Dextrocardia

- Confirm orientation of apex.
- Left-to-right inversion on some fluoroscopy software can be helpful.

Persistent left SVC

- In most cases, the LSVC enters coronary sinus (CS).
- Lead placement from L-side through CS possible.
- Alternative, if right SVC also present, is to implant R-sided device.

AVSD

- If repaired, generally straightforward A-lead and V-lead placement.
- If unrepaired, consider epicardial lead placement at time of concurrent cardiac surgery.
- Surgical patches may make optimal lead placement difficult.
- CS may not be accessible—post-operatively may drain into LA.

1 PACES/HRS Expert Consensus Statement on the Recognition and Management of Arrhythmias in Adult Congenital Heart Disease. Heart Rhythm 2014; 11: e102–e165.

Repaired tetralogy of Fallot
- Generally straightforward lead placement.
- Consider presence of LSVC.
- Significant risk of VT—see section on ICDs.

Ebstein anomaly
- About 4% require pacing.
- RV-lead can be placed into atrialized portion of RV, i.e. above TV.
- Alternative is placement of V-lead into CS, especially after TV surgery to avoid disrupting repaired TV—confirm CS position from operation notes—placement can be below TV.
- Consider epicardial lead placement if concurrent TV surgery is also required.

Post–Mustard or post-Senning operation for TGA
- Accessing the right heart for lead placement usually straightforward unless systemic venous obstruction—baffle stenting may be required.
- Beware baffle leaks—may result in passage of lead into systemic circulation.
- Sub-pulmonary ventricle is morphologically LV and lies to left of midline. Often atrial lead directed towards lateral LA wall—high risk of phrenic nerve stimulation.
- Ideal V-lead position is septal—avoids dyssynchrony and phrenic nerve stimulation.

Univentricular hearts, e.g. Fontan
- Consider vascular access route—e.g. hemi-Fontan, Glenn, Kawashima—may have no access to the right heart from SVC.
- In some cases, an alternative endovascular approach may be necessary, e.g. transhepatic.
- Puncture through an intracardiac baffle/patch may be required, e.g. lateral tunnel Fontan to atrium.
- Consider CS lead placement if on venous side and easily accessible.
- A-lead placement in AP Fontan usually successful.
- V-lead placement can be difficult and may require puncture through baffle/patch to place in systemic circulation—anticoagulation necessary.
- No direct access to heart from venous side in TCPC—requires surgical epicardial lead placement.
- Consider each patient's case individually as variations in anatomy and surgical repair will dictate approach—familiarity with anatomy and previous operations crucial.

Implantable cardiac defibrillators (ICDs)

There is a strong association between complex CHD and SCD. ICD implantation for secondary prevention is recommended by current guidelines (class IB criteria).[2] However, primary prevention criteria is less clear-cut, with most data arising from patients with repaired tetralogy of Fallot.

Insertion of an ICD in younger patients can be associated with significant impact on both lifestyle and morbidity. These include the psychological stress of ICD implantation, such as fear of shocks, risks of lead fracture, repeated generator changes, lifelong infection risk, and impact on quality of life (e.g. sport, driving, occupational restrictions). These factors need to be taken into consideration when deciding on the indication for an ICD, as well as avoiding delay in potentially life-saving therapy. Each case should be discussed in a specialist MDT to achieve consensus opinion.

Special anatomical considerations for ICD insertion

Most of the anatomical considerations are as mentioned in the previous section. However, ICD leads are thicker and more likely to cause perforation. In adults, transvenous leads are widely used. Alternatives include epicardial lead placement (particularly if concurrent cardiac surgery is planned) and subcutaneous ICDs (S-ICD—see following).

Repaired tetralogy of Fallot
- The most-studied groups in terms of risk of SCD and life-threatening VT.
- Indications for ICD are well defined.
- Risk factors for SCD include:
  - NSVT.
  - Previous ventriculotomy.
  - Inducible sustained VT.
  - Elevated LVEDP.
  - Impaired LV systolic function.
  - QRS duration >180 ms.
- ICD therapy well established and placement of leads generally straightforward.

Programming
- Optimal programming requires a balance between appropriate tachycardia therapy and minimal inappropriate shocks.
- Inappropriate shocks often due to atrial arrhythmias with 1:1 conduction. To avoid, consider:
  - Insertion of A-lead.
  - Longer detection times.
  - Use of ATP sequences.
  - Higher HR for VT/VF detection zones.
- Most manufacturer algorithms/discriminators, e.g. PR Logic, not always helpful.

---

2 PACES/HRS Expert Consensus Statement on the Recognition and Management of Arrhythmias in Adult Congenital Heart Disease. Heart Rhythm 2014; 11: e102–e165.

Subcutaneous ICDs

- A subcutaneous device with no intracardiac leads.
- Suitable for patients in whom bradycardia pacing is not required.

Advantages

- Vascular access not required.
- Reduced risk of lead complications.
- Reduced risk of intracardiac infection.
- May avoid need for epicardial lead placement.

Disadvantages

- Bulky device.
- Unable to deliver pacing or ATP therapy—shock-only capability.
- Requires surface ECG mapping to avoid T-wave over-sensing—may preclude many patients with ACHD due to abnormal resting ECGs.
- No data for patients with ACHD.

Cardiac resynchronization therapy (CRT)

There is a paucity of data regarding CRT in adults with repaired congenital heart disease. Conventional adult criteria for CRT cannot always be applied to these patients, e.g. patients with univentricular physiology or a systemic right ventricle. Often there is no LBBB on ECG, making assessment of dyssynchrony by conventional criteria difficult. This is compounded by technical considerations such as unfavourable coronary venous anatomy.

Indications

Often CRT is performed due to pacing-induced heart failure or systemic RV dysfunction. CRT indications in ACHD are mainly class IIa/b by current guidelines.

CRT is not recommended for adults with a QRS duration <120 ms and/or life expectancy <1 year.

Systemic LV
- LVEF ≤35%, SR, NYHA II–IV, LBBB, QRS ≥120 ms.
- LVEF ≤35%, delay transplant/mechanical support.
- LVEF >35%, severe RV dysfunction, NYHA II–IV, RBBB, QRS ≥150 ms.
- LVEF >35%, cardiac surgery, QRS ≥150 ms, progressive LV dilatation/dysfunction.
- V-pacing >40%.

Systemic RV
- RVEF ≤35%, dilated RV, NYHA II–IV, RBBB, QRS ≥150 ms.
- RVEF ≤35%, delay transplant/mechanical support.
- V-pacing >40%.
- TV surgery, NYHA II–IV, RBBB, QRS ≥150 ms.
- RVEF >35%, cardiac surgery, QRS ≥150 ms, progressive RV dilatation/dysfunction.

Single ventricle
- EF ≤35%, ventricular dilatation, NYHA II–IV, QRS ≥150 ms.
- V-pacing >40%.

Anatomical considerations
- Placement of A-lead as described previously.
- V-lead placement can be more difficult—dependent on cardiac anatomy.
- May not always be able to access CS.
- Even if CS accessible, may not allow pacing of systemic ventricle, e.g. atrial switch in TGA.
- Epicardial or hybrid V-lead placement may need to be considered.

Technical considerations for device therapy in ACHD

Pre-procedural planning
- Familiarity with underlying anatomy crucial—obtain previous operation notes, cross-sectional imaging.
  - Is there access into the heart? Some patients (e.g. extracardiac Fontan) will require epicardial pacing.
  - What vessel connects to what?
- Understand the physiology.
  - Risk of systemic emboli in right-to-left shunts.
- Adequate counselling, especially if ICD implant.
- Consider epicardial lead placement if concurrent cardiac surgery planned.
- Consider use of alternative devices, e.g. S-ICD, leadless pacemakers.

Procedural considerations
- Always perform left arm venogram to identify persistent LSVC.
- There may be extensive scar tissue in both the atria and ventricles.
- Choose optimal lead placement site—e.g. avoid RVOT/RV free wall.
- Presence of significant tricuspid or pulmonary regurgitation may make lead implantation difficult.
- Use active fixation leads.
- Consider lead choice, e.g. SelectSecure® leads—smaller size, smaller access sheath, easier extraction, MRI-safe leads.
- If lead in systemic circulation, therapeutic anticoagulation is necessary.
- Consider device depending on indication, e.g. ATP capability if risk of IART, etc.
- Pacemaker programming should minimize risks of V-pacing, e.g. long AV delay, mode switch, etc.

Complications
Due to risks of both short- and long-term complications, placement of pacing/defibrillator devices in young patients requires careful consideration of benefit vs risk. Complications include:
- Repeat procedures for generator changes.
- Infection requiring device extraction and prolonged antibiotics.
- Extraction itself can carry a mortality risk in leads placed >1 year.
- System revision due to lead dislodgement, lead fracture, insulation failure, etc.
- Venous occlusion/thromboembolism.
- Risk of heart failure secondary to V-pacing.
- ICDs—lifestyle and psychological impact, inappropriate shocks.

Contraception and pregnancy

Introduction[1,2,3]

Heart disease is the largest single cause of maternal death in the UK.[4] The number and complexity of survivors of congenital heart disease well enough to consider pregnancy is growing. The maternal risk amongst this population varies from being no different to that of the general population, to carrying a high risk of long-term morbidity and >40% risk of death.

1 Thorne SA, MacGregor AE, Nelson Piercy C. Risk of contraception and pregnancy in heart disease education. 2006; Heart 92: 1520–5.

2 Thorne SA. Pregnancy in heart disease. 2004; Heart 90(4): 450–6.

3 Steer PJ, Gatzoulis MA. (eds). Heart disease and pregnancy (2nd ed.). Cambridge University Press, Cambridge; 2016.

4 Knight M, Kenyon S, Brocklehurst P et al., on behalf of MBRRACE-UK. Saving lives, improving mothers' care—lessons learned to inform future maternity care from the UK and Ireland confidential enquiries into maternal deaths and morbidity, 2009–12. National Perinatal Epidemiology Unit, University of Oxford, Oxford; 2014.

General principles

All adolescent girls and women of childbearing age with congenital heart disease should have access to specialist advice (NB: in this context, 'specialist' = a cardiologist with expertise in both congenital heart disease and cardiac disease in pregnancy, as well as in contraception in heart disease).

Advice should include:
- For the adolescent:
  - Future childbearing potential.
  - Contraceptive options.
- For all women:
  - Awareness of likely maternal risk.
  - Contraception.
- Pre-pregnancy counselling:
  - Maternal risk.
  - Fetal risk.
  - Optimize maternal condition to reduce maternal and fetal risk before pregnancy.
- Antenatal, intrapartum, and post-partum care:
  - In a joint congenital cardiac and obstetric clinic for high-risk conditions.
  - Multidisciplinary team—specialist cardiologist, obstetrician, anaesthetist, haematologist, midwife, congenital cardiac nurse specialist.

Contraception

For the majority of women, contraception is merely a method to conveniently space pregnancies. By contrast, for many women with congenital heart disease, it is a method of preventing a potentially life-threatening condition. Advice should be offered to all females of childbearing age with heart disease.

The cardiovascular safety and contraceptive efficacy of each contraceptive method must be taken into account for each congenital cardiac lesion.

In general, family planning specialists lack expertise in congenital heart disease. The cardiologist must therefore liaise with family planning agencies and have a sound understanding of the risk and efficacy profile of the different contraceptive methods and their suitability for each cardiac lesion.

Contraceptive methods

Barrier methods
- No cardiovascular risk.
- Low efficacy—user dependent.
- Prevents sexually transmitted infection; therefore encourage use in conjunction with other methods.

Oestrogen-containing preparations
- Includes combined oral contraceptive pill (COC), skin patches (vaginal ring and injectable not yet licensed in UK).
- Risk of venous and arterial thromboembolism; therefore contraindicated in many conditions—➔ see Table 21.1.
- Good efficacy.

Progestogen-only methods
- Not prothrombotic, so no hormonal cardiovascular risk. However, may be risk at time of insertion.
- Efficacy varies between methods.
- Menstrual effects vary between methods; all may cause initial irregular bleeding which may be unacceptable. They may be associated with subsequent (reversible) amenorrhoea: an advantage to cyanotic or anticoagulated ♀ in whom menorrhagia is common.

Oral preparations

Standard progestogen-only pill—POP, minipill
- No cardiovascular risk.
- Poor efficacy—do not use in ♀ for whom pregnancy carries significant risk.
- Irregular bleeding may resolve after initial few cycles.

Cerazette/Cerelle®— desogestrel-containing pill
- No cardiovascular risk.
- Efficacy at least as good as COC.
- Irregular bleeding may resolve after initial few cycles.

Table 21.1 Contraindications to COC

Risk of thromboembolism
Dilated cardiac chamberse.g. dilated LA with MV disease, dilated cardiomyopathy
Mechanical valve
Arrhythmia, especially atrial fibrillation
Fontan
PHT—any cause
Previous thromboembolism
Additional risk of paradoxical embolism
Cyanotic heart disease
Unoperated ASD

Long-acting preparations

Depo-Provera®

- No cardiovascular risk, but delivery is by three-monthly deep im injection, so risk of haematoma on warfarin.
- Efficacy good. However, fertility may return rapidly—failure often due to late repeat injections.
- Irregular bleeding may resolve after initial few cycles and be followed by amenorrhoea.

Implanon/Nexplanon®

- Silicon rod inserted subdermally, needs replacing every three years.
- No cardiovascular risk.
- Efficacy better than sterilization.
- Irregular bleeding may be followed by amenorrhoea, but in a few ♀, bleeding is heavy and prolonged, and requires removal of the rod.

Mirena IUS®

- Progestogen-eluting intrauterine device (IUD).
- Cardiovascular risk confined to time of insertion, which should be by a skilled operator, especially for nulliparous ♀.
  - 5% risk of vagal reaction at time of insertion—it is contraindicated in PHT, Fontan circulation, and cyanotic heart disease where a vagal reaction carries a risk of cardiovascular collapse. However, if other methods not acceptable, the risk of insertion by a skilled operator may outweigh the risk of pregnancy.
  - Risk of endocarditis confined to time of insertion. Lower risk than traditional IUD. Current UK guidelines do not recommend antibiotic prophylaxis at insertion.
  - Efficacy better than sterilization.
  - Irregular bleeding often followed by amenorrhoea.

Traditional copper IUD
- Cardiovascular risk as Mirena.
- Efficacy good but less effective than Mirena.
- Painful menorrhagia common.

Sterilization
- Male sterilization rarely appropriate:
  - Assumes monogamy.
  - Man likely to outlive female partner with congenital heart disease.
- Laparoscopic female sterilization:
  - Procedure carries a risk in those for whom pregnancy is the highest risk.
  - Less effective than Mirena and Implanon®.

Preconception

Maternal risks

In order to provide counselling, an up-to-date assessment of the woman's condition and functional capacity is required. Information needed includes thorough history and examination, ECG, echo, and CPEX. Additional information may be needed—24-hour ECG, MRI, cardiac catheterization.

Risks are additive and likely to increase with increasing maternal age, especially for those with complex disease, e.g. with systemic RV. ➔ See Table 21.2.

Canadian risk score for women with pre-existing heart disease[5]
- A useful scoring system for predicting cardiovascular morbidity during pregnancy.
- Four generic risk factors for an adverse cardiovascular event during pregnancy identified in ♀ with pre-existing congenital or acquired heart disease:
  - Cyanosis.
  - NYHA >2.
  - Impaired systemic ventricular function (EF <40%).
  - Previous adverse cardiovascular event.

Physiological response to pregnancy
In the absence of published lesion-specific data, risk can be assessed from whether the heart and circulation are likely to be able to generate the cardiovascular changes that occur in response to pregnancy.
- Lesion-specific risk—➔ see Table 21.3.

Fetal risks
- Any maternal risk.
- Recurrence of congenital heart disease—consider referral for genetic counselling.
  - 50% recurrence for conditions with autosomal dominant inheritance.
  - For most other conditions, risk of recurrence is 4–5%.
  - Risk of recurrence approximately 10% in left heart obstructive lesions, ranging from bicuspid aortic valve to coarctation, Shone complex, and hypoplastic left heart syndrome.
- Maternal cyanosis—chance of livebirth 12% if maternal SaO$_2$ <85%.
- Maternal drugs—e.g. warfarin, angiotensin converting enzyme inhibitors (ACEIs), antiarrhythmics.

Reducing risk pre-pregnancy
- Pre-pregnancy surgery or intervention, e.g.:
  - Aortic valve replacement for AS; consider valve type.
  - Stent relief of coarctation.
  - Arrhythmia ablation.

---

5 Siu SC, Sermer M, Colman JM, et al. (2001). Prospective multicenter study of pregnancy outcomes in women with heart disease. 2001; Circulation 104: 515–21.

Table 21.2 Risk of cardiac event during pregnancy for women with pre-existing heart disease

Number of risk factors present pre-pregnancy	Risk of cardiovascular event in pregnancy
0	5%
1	27%
>1	75%

Table 21.3 Lesion-specific maternal risk—in the absence of other risk factors

Low risk (mortality <1%)	Significant risk (mortality 1–10%)	High risk/contraindicated (mortality >10%)
• Unoperated small or mild:	• Mechanical valve	• PHT
• Pulmonary stenosis	• Systemic RV	• Impaired ventricular function (EF <30%)
• Septal defects	• Cyanosis, no PHT	• Aortic aneurysm
• Patent arterial duct	• Fontan	• Severe L-sided obstruction:
• Most successfully	• Marfan	• MS
repaired:		• AS
• Septal defects		
• Coarctation		
• Tetralogy of Fallot		
• Most regurgitant valve lesions		

NB Risks are additive e.g: MR with LVEF <30% moves to high-risk category. Mechanical valve with systemic RV moves to high-risk category.

NB: *Consider risk of surgery vs reduction in risk of subsequent pregnancy.*
- Timing—early pregnancy may be lower risk for some complex conditions.
- Avoid or accept teratogens, e.g.:
  - Assess functional capacity of ACEI.
  - Discuss fetal and maternal risk of warfarin vs heparin during pregnancy.
  - Continue to take amiodarone but only if it is needed to control non-ablatable life-threatening arrhythmia → accept fetal risk.
- Treat non-cardiac medical conditions, e.g. hypertension, diabetes.
- General measures:
  - Take folic acid.
  - Stop smoking.

Pregnancy and delivery

Detailed discussion of the management of specific conditions is beyond the scope of this text.

Antenatal care

All high significant and high-risk cases (➲ see Table 21.3) should be referred early to a specialist centre for care by the multidisciplinary high-risk team. The frequency of antenatal visits depends on the individual condition and any complications that arise during the pregnancy.

Delivery

In general, spontaneous, normal vaginal delivery carries the lowest haemodynamic maternal risk. Rare cardiac contraindications to vaginal delivery include aortic aneurysm and Marfan with dilated aorta.

A delivery plan including the most appropriate analgesia and the need for invasive monitoring should be documented in the handheld notes. A diagram of the patient's circulation should be included if she has complex disease (e.g. Fontan). The woman and her team need to be prepared to change the plan if maternal or fetal complications develop at any gestational stage.

Post-partum

Post-delivery, high-risk cases should be monitored in an HDU setting for 48 hours. The majority of the cardiovascular changes of pregnancy have resolved by the time of a 6–8-week post-delivery cardiac review, but vigilance is needed to detect and manage any long-term deterioration, especially in ventricular function.

Although not supported by prospective or controlled data, there is concern that ventricular function may not return to normal following delivery in some ♀ with heart disease. In particular, the RV (in ccTGA or TGA post-Mustard or post-Senning) appears to be particularly vulnerable to the volume-loading effects of pregnancy. It may be hypothesized that such patients might benefit from delivery between 36–7 weeks' gestation, to avoid the effects of the last few weeks of volume loading on the ventricle.

Endocarditis

Endocarditis prophylaxis

Nearly all patients with congenital heart disease have a lifelong risk of bacterial endocarditis (Table 22.1) and must be given clear and consistent advice regarding:

- Symptoms that may indicate endocarditis and when to seek expert advice.
- The importance of maintaining good oral hygiene (regular dental review, regular brushing and flossing).
- Up-to-date dental review before any valve surgery or catheter intervention.
- Risk of endocarditis with non-medical procedures, including body piercing and tattoos.

Complex congenital cardiac patients requiring dental surgery under general anaesthetic should be admitted to a specialist centre with collaboration between cardiac anaesthetists, cardiac ICU, maxillofacial surgeons, and adult congenital cardiologists.

Antibiotic prophylaxis

- Current recommendations include UK National Institute for Clinical Excellence (NICE) Guidelines 2008 and European Society of Cardiology Guidelines 2015.
- The lack of concordance between the guidelines reflects the lack of high-level evidence, and physicians should use their clinical judgement about whether any particular guideline should be followed for each individual.
- The importance of good dental hygiene and aseptic technique for procedures remains of utmost importance and should not be allowed to be overshadowed by controversy about antibiotic usage.

UK NICE Guidelines (2008)[1]

- Antibiotic prophylaxis against infective endocarditis is *not* recommended for any patient (Recommendation 1.1.3) for:
  - Dental procedures.
  - Non-dental procedures at upper/lower GI tract; genitourinary, gynaecological, and obstetric procedures including childbirth; upper and lower respiratory tract.
- Any episodes of infection in people at risk of infective endocarditis should be investigated and treated promptly to reduce the risk of endocarditis developing (Recommendation 1.1.5).
- If a person at risk of infective endocarditis is receiving antimicrobial therapy because they are undergoing a GI or GU procedure at a site where there is a suspected infection, the person should receive an antibiotic that covers organisms that cause infective endocarditis (Recommendation 1.1.6).

1 NICE Prophylaxis against infective endocarditis. Clinical Guideline CG64, March 2008. http://www.nice.org.uk/nicemedia/pdf/CG64NICEguidance.pdf

Table 22.1 Risks of developing infective endocarditis or endarteritis in congenital heart disease

Low risk: lesions with no or low velocity turbulence and no prosthetic material

Unoperated	Operated
Anomalous pulmonary venous drainage	Anomalous pulmonary venous drainage
Secundum ASD	Secundum ASD
Ebstein's anomaly	Ebstein's anomaly with repaired native valve
Mild PS	VSD/tetralogy of Fallot without residual lesions
Isolated corrected transposition	PDA
Eisenmenger syndrome without valvar regurgitation	Fontan-type procedures
	Arterial switch for transposition without residual lesions

Moderate risk

Unoperated	Operated
Systemic atrioventricular valve regurgitation	Residual regurgitation of repaired native aortic or systemic atrioventricular valve
Subaortic stenosis	Non-valved conduits
Moderate–severe PS	
Tetralogy of Fallot	

European Society of Cardiology Guidelines (2015)[2]

- Continued use of antibiotic prophylaxis is advised in high-risk patients undergoing high-risk procedures.
- High-risk patients include:
  - Prosthetic valves (including transcathether valves and homografts) and prosthetic material used in valve repair.
  - Patients with previous infective endocarditis.
  - Patients with unrepaired cyanotic heart disease and those who have palliative shunts, conduits, or other prostheses.
- High-risk dental procedures are those that involve periapical or gingival manipulation or perforation of the oral mucosa.

2 ESC Guidelines for the Management of Infective Endocarditis. 2015 Eur Heart J; 36: 3075–3123.

Transition and transfer of care

Transition and transfer of care

Introduction

With the success of paediatric cardiac surgery and intervention over the last 30 years, more children are now surviving into adulthood, particularly those with complex congenital heart defects. Transition describes the process of addressing the specific needs of adolescents and young adults as they move from paediatric-based care towards adult-based care, the end point being the transfer of care to adult health care services. All congenital networks must deliver transition and transfer of care in a manner to minimize the loss of patients, and must take into account the individual's unique needs.

The transition process

- Transition should ideally begin around the start of adolescence, approximately 12 years of age, but needs to be guided by factors such as:
  - Physical development.
  - Psychological development.
  - Emotional maturity.
- There should not be a fixed age of transfer to adult services but should be guided by the young person's readiness, usually 16–19 years of age.
- The views of the young patient must be listened to and considered.
- Families and carers should be involved and supported in discussions.

The transfer process

- The initial appointment in adult services should ideally be in a specialist transfer clinic giving the patient the opportunity to meet their new ACHD consultant and specialist nurse.
- It is important to explore their understanding of their condition and the impact it has on their life, such as:
  - Knowledge of their defect.
  - Symptoms specific to their condition.
  - Career choices they may have.
  - Contraception and pregnancy.
  - Lifestyle issues: smoking, alcohol, recreational drugs, travel.
  - Oral hygiene.
  - What to do in an emergency.
  - Contact details and how to access help.
  - Confidentiality and data protection.
- Age-appropriate information and literature should be readily available for them to read.

The young adult and their family

- Empowering the young person to start to take some responsibility for their own health care is important. Alongside this is the awareness of helping and assisting parents to begin to let their child take a more active role and for them to take a step back. This is not always an easy task, especially with complex patients where the future is less clear.
- This can be a daunting and frightening time for both patient and parent as they leave behind the familiarity of their paediatric team who have cared for them since birth. They now have to put their trust in and develop new relationships with new doctors and nurses. It is not surprising then that some parents can be overprotective, and we must therefore earn their trust and confidence as well as that of our patients.
- Some patients and their parents come as a package or one unit. If the young person wants this to continue, it is important that their ACHD team continue to look after them this way until they have the tools and confidence to make their own decisions. To do otherwise may lead to alienating the young person.

Lifestyle issues

Exercise

Physical activity at an appropriate level has positive effects both on a patient's physical and mental health and should be encouraged in all patients with congenital heart disease.[1]

Many patients with complex heart disease will limit their own activities because of symptoms. Others, however, need guidance to exercise safely.

Exercise for leisure

Type of activity

Fig. 24.1 classifies sport by type (dynamic, static) and intensity (low, moderate, high).[2]
- Dynamic exercise (e.g. walking, jogging):
  - Volume loading with increased cardiac output and O_2 consumption.
  - Modest increase in blood pressure.
  - Suitable for majority of ACHD patients.
- Static exercise (e.g. weightlifting):
  - Pressure loading on the heart.
  - Larger increase in BP, thus not suitable for patients with aortopathy from any cause.
  - Most daily activities include a degree of static exercise.
  - Moderate-to-high intensity types less suitable for many ACHD patients.

Recommendations

Exercise should be discussed regularly with all ACHD patients and risks should be individualized. It is important to take into account their anatomy, any haemodynamically significant residual defects and additional risk factors including arrhythmias, ventricular dysfunction, aortopathy, and elevated pulmonary vascular resistance.

As a guide, the following recommendations can be applied:

Simple lesions without exercise risk factors
- If no or minimal residual disease, no restrictions to type or intensity of exercise performed.

Complex lesions with risk factors
- Avoid high-intensity dynamic and moderate-to-high static exercise.
- If frequent arrhythmias, avoid activities where syncope may be dangerous (e.g. rock climbing).
- Pulmonary hypertension can cause syncope and even sudden cardiac death during any exercise or more than low intensity.
- Activities that risk bodily collision should be avoided in patients with pacemakers or ICDs, recent surgery, or if the patient is anticoagulated.

1 Hirth A, Reybrouck T, Bjarnason-Wehrens B, et al. Recommendations for participation in competitive and leisure sports in patients with congenital heart disease: a consensus document. 2006; Eur J Cardiovasc Prev Rehabil 13(3): 293–9.

2 Pelliccia A, Fagard R, Bjornstad HH, et al. (2005). Recommendations for competitive sports participation in athletes with cardiovascular disease: a consensus document from the Study Group of Sports Cardiology of the Working Group of Cardiac Rehabilitation and Exercise Physiology and the Working Group of Myocardial and Pericardial Diseases of the European Society of Cardiology. 2005; Eur Heart J 26(14): 1422–45.

	A. Low (<40% Max O_2)	**B. Moderate** (40–70% Max O_2)	**C. High** (>70% Max O_2)
III. High (>50% MVC)	Bobsledding/Luge*†, Field events (throwing), Gymnastics*†, Martial arts*, Sailing, Sport climbing, Water skiing*†, Weight lifting*†, Windsurfing*†	Body building*†, Downhill skiing*†, Skateboarding*†, Snowboarding*†, Wresting*	Boxing*, Canoeing, Kayaking, Cycling*†, Decathlon, Rowing, Speed skating*†, Triathlon*†
II. Moderate (20–50% MVC)	Archery, Auto racing*†, Diving*†, Equestrian*†, Motorcycling*†	American football*, Field events (jumping), Figure skating*, Rodeoing*†, Rugby*, Running (sprint), Surfing*†, Synchronized swimming†	Basketball*, Ice hockey*, Cross-country skiing (skating technique), Lacrosse* Running (middle distance), Swimming, Team handball
I. Low (<20% MVC)	Billiards, Bowling, Cricket, Curling, Golf, Riflery	Baseball/Softball*, Fencing, Table tennis, Volleyball	Badminton, Cross-country skiing (classic technique), Field hockey*, Orienteering, Race walking, Racquetball/Squash, Running (long distance), Soccer*, Tennis

Increasing Static Component ←

Increasing Dynamic Component →

Level of exercise: High ▮ High moderate ▮ Moderate ▮ Low moderate ▯ Low ▯

Fig. 24.1 Classification of sports. Classification based on peak static and dynamic components achieved during competition. Higher values may be reached during training.

*Danger of bodily collision.

†† risk if syncope. Reprinted from Mitchell JH, Haskell W, Snell P et al. (2005). Task Force 8: classification of sport. *J Am Coll Cardiol* 45(8), 1313–75 with permission from Elsevier.

Aortopathies

Patients with an aortopathy from any cause are at increased risk of aortic dissection, even if the aortic dimensions are normal. These patients should be advised against static exercise of more than low intensity. This includes patients with connective tissue disorders, bicuspid aortic valve, tetralogy of Fallot, and TGA with arterial switch.

Competitive sport[3]

Pre-participation screening

- Full history (including review of operation note) and examination.
- ECG.
- Echocardiography to assess for residual disease, ventricular function, estimated pulmonary artery pressure.
- Maximal exercise test.

Recommendations

Unrestricted competitive sport only if nil or minimal residual disease.

Follow-up

- Complete reassessment every second to third year.
- Look for unexpected deterioration (ventricular function, regurgitation, arrhythmia).

3 Pelliccia A, Fagard R, Bjornstad HH, et al. (2005). See footnote 2.

Diving

Patients with repaired congenital heart disease are often young and active and may want to participate in activities such as diving.[4] Their suitability for diving needs to be assessed on an individual basis and it is important that they inform the diving company of their underlying condition.

Potential dangers

- Diving reflex:
  - Peripheral vasoconstriction.
  - Fall in heart rate.
- Immersion pulmonary oedema:
  - Rapid increase in systemic vascular resistance during immersion due to overactive vasoconstriction, leading to elevated left atrial pressure and pulmonary oedema.
  - Patients at higher risk if pre-existing ventricular impairment, elevated LA pressure, or significant valvular disease.
- Air embolization—↑ risk if previous chest surgery involving opening of pleura, risk of pathological air trapping.
- Decompression illness—↑ risk if R-to-L shunt.

Cardiovascular requirements for diving

- Normal or near normal exercise capacity.
- Sufficient cardiovascular reserve.
- Absence of R-to-L shunt (or potential R-to-L shunt, e.g. ASD).
  - This is assessed with bubble contract echo including Valsalva.

Specific conditions

Chest surgery

Avoid diving if previous thoracotomy or sternotomy involving pleura (e.g. LIMA graft).

Shunt lesions

- Absolute contraindication to diving if R-L shunt at rest or increased risk of R-L shunt.
- Small and moderate shunts should be assessed on an individual basis, and diving may be possible with careful management of gas load; depth restrictions may apply.

Obstructive valvar lesions

- Diving should be avoided due to patients' inability to increase their cardiac output during the dive.
- Also contraindicated in hypertrophic cardiomyopathy.

Prosthetic valves

- Avoid diving if mechanical valves—risk of bleeding from cuts and bruises due to anticoagulation.
- Diving safe with tissue valves if no significant degeneration.

4 Turner MS. Assessing potential divers with a history of congenital heart disease. Diving and Hyperbaric Medicine 2015; 45(2): 111–15.

Tetralogy of Fallot
- Diving should be avoided if:
  - Reduced exercise capacity.
  - Previous thoracotomy.
  - Residual VSD or significant outflow tract obstruction.
  - Arrhythmia.

Mustard/Senning

Diving contraindicated (abnormal haemodynamic response, risk of arrhythmia and R-to-L shunt from baffle leak).

Other complex congenital heart disease

Diving contraindicated in all cyanotic heart disease and patients with a Fontan circulation.

Travel

Flying

Commercial airplanes all have low ambient cabin pressure, equivalent to altitudes of 5000–8000 m. This leads to a fall in the partial pressure of oxygen and a relative hypoxaemia. This is usually tolerated well with few, if any, symptoms, even in cyanotic patients including Eisenmenger syndrome; supplemental oxygen is rarely needed.[5,6]

Specific precautions for those with limiting disease include:

- Wheelchair/buggy transport within airports to avoid rushing with heavy luggage.
- Keep well hydrated and avoid alcohol during flight.
- DVT prophylaxis—keep mobile and wear anti-thrombosis socks for long-haul flights.
- Break long-haul flights with >24-hour stopover.
- Take letter confirming diagnosis, what to do, and whom to contact in emergency.
- Appropriate travel insurance, including repatriation—*the insurance company must be informed of cardiac condition.*
- The airline should be notified in advance of any significant medical conditions.
- Most airlines will supply in-flight oxygen, although some will charge for this.

Hot climates

- Avoid dehydration.
- Patients with a Fontan circulation particularly at risk of cardiovascular collapse if dehydration occurs.
- Amiodarone therapy can cause severe photosensitivity—advise patients to keep covered up when possible and use high-factor sunblock.

5 Broberg CS, Uebing A, Cuomo L, et al. Adult patients with Eisenmenger syndrome report flying safely on commercial airlines. 2007: Heart 93(12): 1599–1603.

6 Smith D et al. (2010). Fitness to fly for passengers with cardiovascular disease. 2010: Heart 96: ii1–ii16.

Insurance

Patient groups (e.g. The Somerville Foundation in the UK, http://www.thesf.org.uk) are often the most useful source of information to other patients regarding insurance, as companies and premiums will vary enormously.

Travel insurance
- All patients with ACHD should have comprehensive travel insurance whenever they travel.
- The insurance must cover repatriation and emergency medical costs.
- The insurance company must be informed of the patient's cardiac history.
- Premiums vary, but can be prohibitively high for some patients.

Life insurance
- Life insurance is offered on the basis of long-term survival tables.
- Such data is lacking for many congenital cardiac conditions, or is based on outdated surgical and medical practice.
- Many with simple lesions are offered insurance at normal or modestly increased rates.
- Those with complex lesions may be offered insurance at very high rates or turned down altogether. Such individuals should seek advice from patient groups or independent brokers before applying.

Insurance

Travel Insurance

Life insurance

Glossary of terms

Aortography Contrast radiography of aorta to demonstrate abnormalities of the aortic valve, ascending aorta, aortic arch, and descending aorta.

Atresia Congenital or acquired condition in which a valve or artery fails to develop, leaving severe stenosis or complete occlusion, e.g. pulmonary or tricuspid atresia.

Atrial septal defect Defect in wall between atria.

Baffle Surgically created wall within the atrial mass, for instance in Mustard/Senning or Fontan operations.

Coarctation Narrowing in aorta, typically in the post-ductal region, but can involve aortic arch.

Conduit Surgically created tube connection, can be valved, between two vascular channels, e.g. Fontan extracardiac conduit with no valve or valved RV–PA conduit.

Cor triatriatum Membrane within the left atrium.

Cyanosis Arterial saturation <95%

Dacron® Artificial material used to close defects, create conduits and baffles.

Double outlet right ventricle (DORV) Condition where both great arteries arise from the right ventricle.

Down syndrome Trisomy 21.

Ebstein anomaly Abnormality of right heart caused by failure of delamination of tricuspid valve leaflets leading to apical displacement of the valve and atrialization of the right ventricle.

Erythrocytosis Increased numbers of red blood cells, often as a result of systemic desaturation.

Fontan operation Palliative surgery for univentricular hearts, first performed by Francis Fontan.

Functionally univentricular heart The heart has unequal-sized ventricles making biventricular circulation not possible.

Gadolinium® Contrast agent used in magnetic resonance imaging of the heart.

Gore-Tex® Artificial material used to close defects, create conduits and baffles.

Hypoplastic left heart syndrome (HLHS) Condition characterized by failure to develop left heart structures, leaving a functionally univentricular heart, with a small left ventricle, small mitral valve, small aorta, and aortic arch.

Intra-atrial reentrant tachycardia (IART) Scar-related atypical atrial flutter, common in operated congenital heart defects, particularly dangerous post–Fontan, Mustard, and Senning surgery.

Mustard/Senning procedure (operation) Palliative surgery for simple transposition in which the systemic and pulmonary venous returns are redirected by means of an intra-atrial baffle to relieve cyanosis. Now superseded by the arterial switch operation.

Patent ductus arteriosus (PDA) Persistence of the fetal arterial duct beyond the neonatal period.

Patent foramen ovale Persistence of the foramen ovale beyond the neonatal period, present in around 25% of the adult population.

Protein-losing enteropathy Condition in which there is persistent loss of protein through the GI tract, characterized by low serum albumin and chronic pleural effusions, ascites and dependent oedema, and high faecal alpha1-antitrypsin levels. Carries a poor prognosis.

Pulmonary arteriography Contrast radiography of the pulmonary circulation.

Pulmonary atresia Absence of the pulmonary valve/artery in development, occasionally acquired following severe pulmonary valvar of subvalvar stenosis.

Pulmonary hypertension Elevation of the mean pulmonary arterial pressure above 25 mmHg at rest or 35 mmHg on exercise; can be idiopathic or acquired.

Radical repair Term used to describe surgical correction of tetralogy of Fallot, with resection of the RVOT muscle bundles and patch closure of the VSD ± transannular patch.

Scimitar syndrome Anomalous venous drainage of right lung with anomalous vein passing below the diaphragm to enter into the IVC, with typical 'scimitar' shadow on CXR. Often associated with sequestered right lower lobe, with arterial supply from descending aorta.

Shone complex (syndrome) Syndrome characterized by multiple left-sided obstructive lesions, such as mitral stenosis, subvalvar and valvar aortic stenosis, hypoplastic aortic arch and coarctation of the aorta.

Shunt Connection between two blood vessels aimed at increasing blood flow to the distal vessel, e.g. Blalock-Taussig shunt.

Sternotomy Midline incision through the sternum to allow access to the heart and great vessels.

Tetralogy of Fallot Commonest cyanotic heart defect, characterized by anterior superior deviation of the interventricular septum, leading to a VSD, RVOTO, RVH, and aortic override.

Thoracotomy Lateral incision in the chest wall to allow access to the pulmonary arteries, aortic arch, subclavian vessels, and mitral valve.

Transposition of the great arteries Condition in which ventriculoarterial discordance is present, i.e. the right ventricle leads to the aorta and the left ventricle to the pulmonary artery.

Valvuloplasty Opening of stenosed valve by means of surgical incision or balloon dilatation.

Venesection The removal of one unit of blood to alleviate the symptoms of hyperviscosity in cyanotic heart disease.

Ventricular septal defect (VSD) Defect in the wall separating the two ventricles.

Wood unit Unit of vascular resistance named after the pioneering cardiologist Paul Wood. 1 wood unit is approximately 80 dyne.sec/cm^5.

List of operations for congenital heart disease

Arterial switch

- Corrective operation for TGA (usually as neonate).
- Great arteries switched over and re-anastomosed to establish VA concordance. Coronaries reimplanted to neo-aorta (formerly pulmonary trunk).
- Restores LV to systemic circulation.
- Brings PAs to lie anterior to the aorta (LeCompte manoeuvre).

Atrioventricular septal defect repair

- Atrial and ventricular septation using one or two patches, partitioning of common AV valve into left and right AV valves.
- Left AV valve repair—usually closure of 'cleft' formed from approximation of superior and inferior bridging leaflets to form 'anterior' leaflet of left AV valve.
- Late reoperation typically required for recurrent left AV valve regurgitation/ LVOT obstruction.

Bentall procedure (aortic root replacement)

- Used in aortic root dilatation, aortoannular ectasia, ascending aortic (AA) aneurysm, and type A dissection that involves the valve.
- AA and AV replaced by a composite graft (i.e. a tube graft with an AV already sewn into it).
- Coronary arteries reimplanted into the side of conduit.

Blalock-Hanlon atrial septectomy (historical)

- Palliative or staging procedure previously used in TGA.
- ASD created via surgical approach (R thoracotomy) without cardiopulmonary bypass.
- Allows mixing of systemic and pulmonary circulations at atrial level to improve arterial saturations.

Blalock-Taussig shunt

- Palliative or staging shunt to increase pulmonary blood flow in pulmonary atresia or PS, e.g. tetralogy of Fallot. Often referred to as an arterial shunt or a systemic-pulmonary shunt (to differentiate from venous shunts/connections).
- Classical Blalock-Taussig (historical)—direct anastomosis between subclavian artery and ipsilateral PA.
- Modified Blalock-Taussig—Gore-Tex® tube graft used between subclavian (or innominate) and PAs.
- Can be L- or R-sided and performed via a thoracotomy or midline sternotomy.

Brock procedure (historical)

- Palliative procedure to increase pulmonary blood flow and decrease R-to-L shunt in tetralogy of Fallot.
- Resection of RV infundibular muscle through an RV incision.
- Performed without cardiopulmonary bypass through either a midline sternotomy or a left anterior thoracotomy.

Coarctation repair

- Coarctation segment is excised and the aortic ends re-anastomosed.
- Occasionally the narrowed segment is enlarged using either a synthetic patch or the divided left subclavian artery.
- Usually performed via thoracotomy. Sternotomy and CPB if significant transverse arch hypoplasia.

Damus-Kaye-Stansel operation

- Direct anastomosis of the main PA to the aorta to create a single, conjoint arterial outlet from the heart (the main PA is separated from the branch PAs which must be supplied by a shunt or conduit).
- Usually reserved for functionally univentricular circulations to produce an unobstructed systemic outflow in complex aortic and subaortic stenosis/hypoplasia.
- Occasionally used in biventricular repair, baffling VSD through to the neo-aorta and placing an RV–PA conduit (see Yasui procedure).

Double-switch operation

- Corrective procedure for ccTGA.
- Arterial and atrial switch (see Mustard and Senning procedure).
- Restores the morphological LV to the systemic circulation ('anatomical repair').
- Only possible if the LV is trained preoperatively to work against systemic resistance.

Ebstein anomaly repair

- Modern repair aims to reposition tricuspid valve to anatomical annulus in a spiral fashion ('cone repair').
- Traditional approaches involve replacement or repair by monocuspidization/ bicuspidization of tricuspid valve and plication of annulus/ventricularized atrium. Rarely in neonate—tricuspid valve closure and shunt (Starnes procedure).

Fontan procedure

- Definitive palliative procedure for functionally univentricular hearts, e.g. tricuspid atresia, double inlet LV, hypoplastic L heart.
- Usually preceded by Glenn (cavopulmonary) anastomosis.
- Fontan circulation—IVC and SVC connected directly to PAs. Blood flow though the lungs relies on passive flow (no ventricle) down a venous pressure gradient.
- Pulmonary and systemic circulations are separated (i.e. acyanotic circulation *but* many incorporate a fenestration that allows for a small R–L shunt).
- Classic Fontan—direct anastomosis between RA and PA (called atriopulmonary connection).
- Total cavopulmonary connection (TCPC)—both the IVC and SVC are connected individually into the PAs using a bidirectional Glenn for the SVC and either:
  - Lateral tunnel TCPC—within the RA between IVC and RPA, or
  - Extracardiac Fontan—IVC ↓ PA via extracardiac Gore-Tex® conduit.

Glenn shunt

- Palliative or staging shunt to increase pulmonary blood flow (low pressure) in pulmonary atresia or severe stenosis to increase arterial saturations.
- Classic Glenn (historical)—SVC end-to-end anastomosis with the divided RPA (often via R thoracotomy).
- Bidirectional Glenn—end-to-side anastomosis of divided SVC to the undivided PA (bidirectional implies flow to both lungs). Also called a 'cavopulmonary shunt'.
- Characterized by late development of arteriovenous fistulae in the lung(s) supplied by the Glenn.

Interrupted aortic arch repair

- Interruption segment excised and proximal/distal aorta mobilized, ends re-anastomosed.
- Anastomosis often augmented using a patch (typically pulmonary artery homograft).
- Right subclavian artery occasionally sacrificed if aberrant.

Kawashima operation (two meanings)

- 1. The name is most typically used for a Glenn shunt in the setting of azygous continuation of the IVC (usually L isomerism). Thus, the procedure shunts both the SVC and IVC blood to the lungs (effectively a Fontan circulation except that the hepatic veins still drain to the RA).
- 2. Also used for a corrective procedure for some types of DORV—intracardiac tunnelling of the VSD through to the aorta.

Konno operation

- Corrective operation for tunnel-type subvalvar AS.
- LVOT enlarged with patch, applied through a right ventriculotomy. May be combined with AV replacement.
- Commonly performed in conjunction with a Ross procedure ('Ross-Konno').

Mustard procedure and Senning procedure

- Definitive palliative operations for TGA (atrial switch procedures). RV still supports systemic circulation and LV the pulmonary circulation.
- Mustard—atrial baffle created from pericardium or synthetic material.
- Senning—only uses native tissue to create the baffle.
- Baffle directs systemic venous return to LV and pulmonary venous return to RV.

Norwood procedure (staged palliation for HLHS)

- Stage I—Neonatal operation (single-ventricle repair) combining Damus-Kaye-Stansel anastomosis and aortic arch repair utilizing the RV as the systemic ventricle and creating a systemic shunt to supply the pulmonary circulation. Can be either an aortopulmonary shunt or RV–PA (Sano) shunt.
- Stage II (4–10 months)—bidirectional Glenn to replace systemic shunt.
- Stage III (2–4 years)—completion of Fontan circulation.

Potts shunt (historical)

- Palliative shunt to increase pulmonary blood flow in PS or pulmonary atresia.
- Descending aorta ↓ LPA direct anastomosis. Difficult to control flow; sometimes caused pulmonary vascular disease.
- Usually performed via L thoracotomy.

PA banding

- Palliative or staging procedure to protect lungs from high flow or pressure.
- Can be used with a view to subsequent corrective surgery—e.g. in neonate with multiple VSDs.
- More commonly used in functionally single-ventricle circulations with unrestricted pulmonary blood flow.
- Effectively it is surgically created PS.
- Also used in TGA/ccTGA for LV 'training' if considering late switch or double switch.

Pulmonary atresia/VSD with MAPCAs

- Unifocalization during early years of life to join important MAPCAs to central pulmonary arteries with creation of an RV–PA conduit or creation of an aortopulmonary shunt to encourage growth of native PAs.
- Complete repair (VSD closure and placement of RV–PA conduit) if adequate supply to both lungs by combination of main PAs and unifocalized vessels.

Rashkind procedure

- Staging balloon atrial septostomy in neonates to allow mixing of systemic and pulmonary circulations in TGA prior to definitive surgery.

Rastelli procedure

- Corrective operation for TGA + VSD + PS.
- VSD closed with patch that is used to connect the LV to the anterior aorta.
- RV to PA conduit.
- Term is frequently incorrectly applied to any procedure involving an RV–PA conduit. It should be reserved for TGA/VSD/PS.
- A Rastelli-Senning operation is a combined atrial switch with Rastelli for ccTGA with a large VSD and PS or pulmonary atresia.

Ross procedure

- Aortic valve replacement using pulmonary autograft.
- Homograft pulmonary valve replacement.

Senning procedure

➔ See Mustard procedure and Senning procedure, p. 234.

Tetralogy of Fallot repair
- Patch closure of VSD.
- Relief of RVOT obstruction—resection of RV infundibular muscle. ± patch to enlarge main/ branch PA's ± RVOT (transannular patch if PV inadequate).
- Monocusp valve sometimes created in setting of transannular patch to maintain (often) short-term PV competence.
- RV–PA conduit required on occasion for major coronary artery crossing RVOT or very small PAs.

Truncus arteriosus repair
- Corrective surgery in neonatal period.
- Pulmonary arteries detached from trunk and joined to RV via valved conduit.
- VSD patch closure.
- Truncal valve repair may be required for incompetence.

Valve-sparing aortic root replacement
- Procedure of choice for young patients requiring aortic root replacement with well-functioning aortic valve.
- The aortic root is replaced using a synthetic graft (Dacron) and the native aortic valve reimplanted within it.
- Alternative to Bentall procedure.

Waterston shunt (historical)
- Palliative systemic-pulmonary shunt for severe PS or atresia to increase pulmonary blood flow.
- AA ↓ RPA direct anastomosis. Difficult to control flow, sometimes caused pulmonary vascular disease.
- Often performed via R thoracotomy.

Yasui procedure
- Combination of Norwood and Rastelli procedures.
- Used for complex LVOT obstruction with a VSD and adequate left ventricle.
- Can be performed as a single-stage neonatal procedure or as a staged procedure, with Norwood stage I in neonatal period, followed by Rastelli biventricular repair with RV–PA conduit at around 8–12 months of age.

Common valve and conduit types

An exhaustive list of all commercially available prosthetic valves and conduits are beyond the scope of this chapter. The most commonly used in the current era, as well as some widely used during earlier years, are listed.

Prosthetic heart valves

Mechanical heart valves

Mechanical heart valves are a popular choice for aortic and mitral valve replacement in young adults due to superior durability over bioprosthetic valves. All require full anticoagulation.

Bi-leaflet tilting disk valves

- The most widely used mechanical valve due to haemodynamic profile and durability.
- Durability: greater than 94% freedom from reoperation at 20 years.
- Common examples: St Jude bi-leaflet, Sorin Carbomedics, Medtronic ATS.
- The newer On-X mechanical valve has a flared subvalvar inflow guard which may prevent pannus in-growth and may require lower levels of anticoagulation (trial results awaited).

Earlier generation mechanical valves

- Rarely implanted now due to poorer haemodynamic profile and durability.
- Single tilting disk: Medtronic-Hall, Bjork-Shiley, Lillehei-Kaster, Omnicarbon.
- Ball-in-cage: Starr-Edwards.

Bioprosthetic heart valves

- A popular choice for aortic and mitral valve replacement in older adults where valve durability is less important, and in younger patients where anticoagulation is contraindicated or undesirable.
- In the aortic position, freedom from structural valve deterioration (SVD) is around 85% at 10 years and 52% at 20 years in patients less than 60 years of age at implant, and full anticoagulation is not needed.
- Freedom from SVD (requiring replacement) in the mitral position in patients younger than 60 years at implant declines from >85% at 10 years to 57% at 15 years.
- Earlier degeneration seen in young patients, presumed to be due to higher activity levels and calcium turnover.
- Popular choice for pulmonary and tricuspid valve replacement, with excellent durability (76% freedom from SVD at 15 years).
- Possibility of subsequent valve-in-valve percutaneous valve replacement (not possible with mechanical valves).

Stented Xenograft pericardial valves

- Porcine, equine, or bovine pericardial tissue mounted in a polyester-covered metal stent with sewing ring.
- Examples: Carpentier-Edwards Perimount, St Jude Trifecta, St Jude Epic, Sorin Pericarbon.
- The Sorin Mitroflow valve has demonstrated early calcification and rapid structural deterioration in some young patients.
- Popular choice for pulmonary valve replacement with good durability in this position.

Stentless Xenograft pericardial valves
- Pericardial valve mounted on a small sewing ring but with no struts or stent to support the leaflets.
- Commissures are suspended surgically to the aortic sinus, theoretically maximizing valve opening area and haemodynamic profile.
- Examples: Sorin Freedom, ATS 3F.

Stent-mounted Xenograft pericardial valves
- Bovine pericardial valves pre-mounted within a nitinol stent for transcatheter aortic valve replacement (Medtronic CoreValve, Edwards SAPIEN, St Jude Portico) or rapid surgical aortic valve replacement (Sorin Perceval).
- Increasingly used for transcutaneous pulmonary valve replacement within an existing conduit.

Xenograft aortic valves
- Porcine aortic valves mounted on a stent of polypropylene or metal alloy with a silicone sewing ring covered in polyester fabric.
- Common types: Medtronic Hancock/Mosaic, Carpentier-Edwards, St Jude Epic.

Other
- Dura mater/fascia lata valves now rarely used.

Autologous valves
- The pulmonary valve used as an autograft to replace the aortic or (less commonly) the mitral valve (Ross procedure).
- Popular in children because of the possibility of growth in the autograft and no need for anticoagulation.
- Autologous valves have also been constructed from glutaraldehyde-fixed autologous pericardium. Long-term durability remains uncertain.

Valved conduits

Mechanical valved conduits

- Most commonly used in replacement of the aortic root (Bentall procedure), one of the aforementioned mechanical valve prostheses is sewn into a woven polyester tube.

Biological valved conduits

Homografts

- Human aortic and pulmonary valves harvested from donors where the entire heart is not suitable for transplantation.
- The conduit is preserved by fixation and/or cyro-preservation.
- Very commonly used in congenital cardiac surgery because of the ease of use and wide range of available sizes.
- Limited availability.
- Most commonly used in the aortic position in the treatment of infective endocarditis with root abscess, and in the reconstruction of the right ventricular outflow tract/pulmonary valve replacement in a wide range of conditions.

Bovine jugular vein (Medtronic Contegra, Venpro)

- Glutaraldehyde-preserved valved bovine jugular vein.
- Available in a range of sizes from 12 mm to 22 mm.
- Often used for RV–PA conduit if a suitable homograft not available.
- Durability similar to homograft in small patients, but with a higher rate of late endocarditis.

Stent-mounted bovine jugular vein (Melody valve)

- Bovine jugular vein pre-mounted in a balloon-expandable stent.
- Allows percutaneous replacement of the pulmonary valve within the annular ring of a bio-prosthesis, or after pre-stenting of homograft/ xenograft conduits.

Composite synthetic/bioprosthetic conduits

- A commercially available porcine valve within a synthetic polyester conduit commonly used as a right ventricle to pulmonary artery conduit (Medtronic Hancock or Carpentier-Edwards conduit).
- Custom-valved conduits can also be created from Gelweave Dacron conduit material and either pericardial or aortic valve xenografts.

Porcine root xenograft (Medtronic Freestyle)

- Less widely used, the glutaraldehyde-preserved porcine aortic root has been used as an aortic root replacement substitute, and also as an RV–PA conduit in adult-size patients when a suitable homograft is not available.

List of syndromes

List of syndromes and their associations

Table A3.1 Table of syndromes and their associations

Syndrome	Chromosomal defect	Cardiac defects	Key non-cardiac features	Key facial features
Alagille	20p12 jagged gene (AD)	PS, pulmonary artery stenosis	Hypoplasia of hepatic ducts, hepatocellular carcinoma.	Broad forehead, pointed chin, long bulbous nose
Cat eye	22q11 duplication	TAPVD	Renal and bowel anomalies	Coloboma
Cri du Chat	Deletion 5p	VSD, ASD, PDA, tetralogy of Fallot	Low IQ, growth retardation, high-pitched cry	Round face, flat nose, micrognathia
DiGeorge (CATCH 22)	Deletion 22q11	Tetralogy of Fallot, interrupted aortic arch, truncus arteriosus, DORV	Immunodeficiency, cleft palate low IQ, behavioural and psychiatric disorders	Micrognathia, low-set ears, cleft palate, short philtrum
Down	Trisomy 21	AVSD, VSD, MVP	Low IQ, hypothyroidism, dementia	Upslanting palpebral fissures, tongue protrusion
Edwards	Trisomy 18	VSD, PS, and AS	Low IQ, severe growth retardation. Majority die in 1st year.	Small eyes, short nose, micrognathia
Ellis-van Creveld	4p16 (AR)	Common atrium, VSD, ASD, PDA	Thoracic dysplasia, disproportionate dwarfism, 50% die in infancy	Abnormal teeth, sparse hair, 'lip tie'
Holt-Oram	12q2 (AD)	ASD, VSD	Upper limb abnormalities	
Marfan	Fibrillin gene defect (AD)	Aortic root dilation, MVP	Joint disorders, pneumothorax	Lens dislocation, high arch palate
Noonan	12q24 (AD)	PS, HCM	Short stature, bleeding disorders	Triangular face, low hair line, webbed neck

(Continued)

Table A3.1 (Contd.)

Syndrome	Chromosomal defect	Cardiac defects	Key non-cardiac features	Key facial features
Turner	XO	Bicuspid aortic valve, coarctation, anomalies of systemic and pulmonary venous drainage	Infertile (unless mosaic), osteoporosis, renal anomalies	Similar phenotype to Noonan syndrome
William	Multi-gene deletion 7q11	Supravalvar AS, hypoplastic aorta, PS	Low IQ, hypercalcaemia	Elfin facies— wide mouth, full cheeks, small chin,
Wolf-Hirschhorn	Deletion 4p	ASD, VSD, persistent LSVC	Low IQ, growth retardation. 1/3 die in infancy	'Greek warrior helmet' face

Further reading

Gorlin RJ, Cohen MM, Hennekam RCM. Syndromes of the head and neck (4th ed.). Oxford University Press, Oxford; 2001.

Online Mendelian Inheritance in Man (OMIM™). ℘ http://www.nslij-genetics.org/search_omim. html.

Index

implantable cardiac
defibrillators 204–5
procedural
considerations 207
pre-procedural
planning 207
dextrocardia, bradycardia
pacing 202
DiGeorge syndrome (dele-
tion 22q11) 252
diving 232–3
double-chambered right
ventricle 90
double inlet left
ventricle 162
post-Fontan
operation 167
double orifice mitral
valve 86
double-switch
operation 243
Down syndrome (trisomy
21) 252
atrioventricular septal
defects 108–9
ductus arteriosus 64
dynamic exercise 228, 229

E

Ebstein anomaly 9, 92–5
bradycardia pacing 203
chest X-ray 22
endocarditis risk 221
transthoracic echocardiography 93, 94
Ebstein anomaly repair 243
echocardiography
transoesophageal 28–30
transthoracic 26–7
Edwards syndrome (trisomy
18) 252
Eisenmenger syndrome 9,
39, 112–13
chest X-ray 23
endocarditis risk 221
see also pulmonary arterial
hypertension
Ellis–van Creveld
syndrome 252
emergencies 190
in cyanotic heart
disease 190
haemoptysis in a cyanotic
patient 190
haemoptysis or haema-
temesis in patients
with repaired
coarctation 191
tachyarrhythmias 192–4
endocarditis
prophylaxis 220–1

European Society
of Cardiology
Guidelines 221
UK NICE
guidelines 220–1
endocarditis risks,
lesion-specific 221
end-of-life care 198
endothelin
antagonists 180, 197
epidemiology 4
exercise 228–30
and aortopathies 230
classification of sports 229
competitive sport 230
exercise testing 42
cardiopulmonary 44–5
types of tests 43

F

fetal circulation 64
flying 234
Fontan circulation
atrial tachyarrhyth-
mias 192–3
bradycardia pacing 203
cardiac catheterization 50
cardiac MR 36
catheter interventions 59
DC cardioversion 193
diving 233
endocarditis risk 221
failure of 172–3
general principles 166
heart failure 197
hot climates 234
maternal pregnancy
risk 217
transoesophageal
echocardiography 29
Fontan procedure 164,
165, 243
long-term
complications 169, 171
long-term outcome 173
post-surgery
assessment 166–9
post-surgery
management 170
surgical approaches 166
foramen ovale 64
patent 102–3
functionally univentricular
heart 160
bradycardia pacing 203
Damus–Kaye–Stansel
procedure 243
Fontan procedure 243
staged surgical
approach 164
see also Fontan procedure

G

gadolinium contrast 32
general anaesthesia, post-
Fontan patients 170
genetic counselling 216
Ghent criteria, Marfan
syndrome 124
Glenn operation (cavo-
pulmonary shunt) 67,
69, 164, 165, 244
great arteries, description
of 10–12

H

haematemesis, in
patients with repaired
coarctation 191
haematocrit, elevated 74
haemoptysis 77
in a cyanotic patient 190
in patients with repaired
coarctation 191
heart (heart-lung)
transplantation 198
heart failure 196
drug therapy 197
end-of-life care 198
transplantation 198
Holt–Oram
syndrome 99, 252
homograft valved
conduits 243
hypoplastic left heart syndrome (HLHS) 174, 175
Norwood procedure 244

I

imaging, non-invasive 18
cardiovascular mag-
netic resonance
imaging 32–6
chest X-ray 20–4
computed
tomography 38–9
transoesophageal echo
(TOE) 28–30
transthoracic
echocardiography 26–7
Implanon® 213
implantable cardiac defibrillators (ICDs) 204–5
complications 207
subcutaneous 205
technical
considerations 207
incremental shuttle walk
test 43
inferior vena cava
anomalies 129